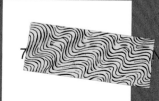

ARTERIAL
BLOOD GASES
MADE EASY

Arterial Blood Gases Made Easy

Second Edition

Iain A M Hennessey MBChB (Hons) BSc (Hons) MMIS FRCS

Consultant Paediatric Surgeon and Clinical Lead for Innovation, Alder Hey Children's Hospital, Liverpool, UK

Alan G Japp MBChB (Hons) BSc (Hons) MRCP PhD

Consultant Cardiologist, Royal Infirmary of Edinburgh and St John's Hospital, Livingston, UK

ELSEVIER

Edinburgh   London   New York   Oxford   Philadelphia   St Louis   Sydney   Toronto   2016

ELSEVIER

First edition 2007
Second edition 2016

ISBN   9780702061905
International ISBN   9780702061912

British Library Cataloguing in Publication Data
A catalogue record for this book is available from the British Library

Library of Congress Cataloging in Publication Data
A catalog record for this book is available from the Library of Congress

Notices
Knowledge and best practice in this field are constantly changing. As new research and experience broaden our understanding, changes in research methods, professional practices, or medical treatment may become necessary.

Practitioners and researchers must always rely on their own experience and knowledge in evaluating and using any information, methods, compounds, or experiments described herein. In using such information or methods they should be mindful of their own safety and the safety of others, including parties for whom they have a professional responsibility.

With respect to any drug or pharmaceutical products identified, readers are advised to check the most current information provided (i) on procedures featured or (ii) by the manufacturer of each product to be administered, to verify the recommended dose or formula, the method and duration of administration, and contraindications. It is the responsibility of practitioners, relying on their own experience and knowledge of their patients, to make diagnoses, to determine dosages and the best treatment for each individual patient, and to take all appropriate safety precautions.

To the fullest extent of the law, neither the publisher nor the authors, contributors, or editors, assume any liability for any injury and/or damage to persons or property as a matter of products liability, negligence or otherwise, or from any use or operation of any methods, products, instructions, or ideas contained in the material herein.

Content Strategist: Laurence Hunter
Content Development Specialist: Helen Leng
Project Manager: Louisa Talbott
Designer: Christian Bilbow
Illustration Manager: Amy Naylor
Illustrator: Graeme Chambers; Jade Myers of Matrix and Vicky Heim

Contents

Contents

Preface

If you've taken the time to open *Arterial Blood Gases Made Easy*, you must believe that arterial blood gases (ABGs) are important, but not entirely straightforward.

We certainly agree on the first point: ABG analysis now plays an indispensable role in the assessment and management of patients with a huge range of acute medical and surgical problems. On the second point, we hope our book can be of assistance.

For this second edition of *Arterial Blood Gases Made Easy* we have remained true to our original principles of avoiding extraneous detail and focusing on the aspects of ABG analysis that are practical and useful. In this spirit we have been sparing with our additions to Part 1 of the book but have added 5 new clinical scenarios to Part 2 and included a new video showing how to obtain an arterial sample. We continue to believe that many medical and nursing students, junior doctors and specialist nurses will benefit from a clear, concise guide to performing and interpreting ABGs.

Iain A M Hennessey
Alan G Japp

Acknowledgements

We are indebted to Dr J K Baillie for his advice, suggestions and constructive criticism. We would also like to thank Heather Milne for allowing us to film her wrists for the demonstration video. Finally, we are grateful to Laurence Hunter and Helen Leng for their unfailing support and patience.

INTRODUCTION

Arterial blood gas (ABG) analysis refers to the measurement of pH and the *partial pressures* of oxygen (O_2) and carbon dioxide (CO_2) in arterial blood. From these values we can assess the state of *acid–base balance* in blood and how well lungs are performing their job of *gas exchange*.

Already there are questions: What is meant by 'acid–base status'? What is a 'partial pressure'? Why do they matter? It helps to break things down.

Part 1 of this book is designed to answer these questions. We start with a few pages covering the basic essentials of respiratory and acid–base physiology: *please do not skip them!* If you understand these core concepts, the rest will follow seamlessly. Part 1 also explains how, when, and why to obtain an ABG sample, before concluding with a simple step-by-step guide for interpreting ABG data.

Part 2 then allows you to put all of this into practice with a series of case scenarios involving ABG analysis. You may already have a method for interpreting ABGs but we urge you to try our system (set out in Section 1.9) that offers a logical, methodical and consistent way of approaching ABGs. By seeing how this system can identify all of the major patterns of ABG abnormalities, we hope you will gain the necessary confidence to apply it in clinical practice.

PULMONARY GAS EXCHANGE: THE BASICS

Our cells use oxygen (O_2) to generate energy and produce carbon dioxide (CO_2) as waste. Blood supplies cells with the O_2 they need and clears the unwanted CO_2. This process depends on the ability of our lungs to enrich blood with O_2 and rid it of CO_2.

Pulmonary gas exchange refers to the transfer of O_2 from the atmosphere to the bloodstream (oxygenation) and CO_2 from the bloodstream to the atmosphere (CO_2 elimination).

The exchange takes place between tiny air sacs called *alveoli* and blood vessels called *capillaries*. Because they each have extremely thin walls and come into very close contact (the alveolar–capillary membrane), CO_2 and O_2 are able to move (*diffuse*) between them (Figure 1).

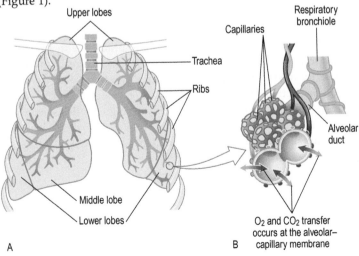

Upper lobes

Trachea

Ribs

Middle lobe

Lower lobes

A

Capillaries

Respiratory bronchiole

Alveolar duct

O_2 and CO_2 transfer occurs at the alveolar–capillary membrane

B

Figure 1 *Respiratory anatomy.*

PULMONARY GAS EXCHANGE: PARTIAL PRESSURES

Arterial blood gases (ABGs) help us to assess the effectiveness of gas exchange by providing measurements of the *partial pressures* of O_2 and CO_2 in arterial blood (i.e. the PaO_2 and $PaCO_2$).

Partial pressure describes the contribution of one individual gas within a gas mixture (such as air) to the total pressure. When a gas dissolves in liquid (e.g. blood), the amount dissolved depends on the partial pressure.

Note

PO_2 = **partial pressure of O_2**
PaO_2 = **partial pressure of O_2 in *arterial blood***

Gases move from areas of higher partial pressure to lower partial pressure. At the alveolar–capillary membrane, air in alveoli has a higher PO_2 and lower PCO_2 than capillary blood. Thus, O_2 molecules move from alveoli to blood and CO_2 molecules move from blood to alveoli until the partial pressures are equal.

A note on ... gas pressures

At sea level, atmospheric pressure (i.e. total pressure of gases in the atmosphere) = 101 kPa or 760 mmHg.

O_2 comprises 21% of air, so the partial pressure of O_2 in air
= 21% of atmospheric pressure
= 21 kPa or 160 mmHg

CO_2 makes up just a tiny fraction of air, so the partial pressure of CO_2 in inspired air is negligible.

CARBON DIOXIDE ELIMINATION

Diffusion of CO_2 from the bloodstream to alveoli is so efficient that CO_2 elimination is actually limited by how quickly we can 'blow off' the CO_2 in our alveoli. Thus, the Pa_{CO_2} (which reflects the overall amount of CO_2 in arterial blood) is determined by *alveolar ventilation* – the total volume of air transported between alveoli and the outside world every minute.

Ventilation is regulated by an area in the brainstem called the *respiratory centre*. This area contains specialised chemical receptors that sense the Pa_{CO_2} and connect with the muscles involved in breathing. If it is abnormal, the respiratory centre adjusts the rate and depth of breathing accordingly (Figure 2).

Normally, lungs can maintain a normal Pa_{CO_2}, even in conditions where CO_2 production is unusually high (e.g. sepsis). Consequently, an increased Pa_{CO_2} (hypercapnia) virtually always implies reduced alveolar ventilation.

Key point

Pa_{CO_2} is controlled by ventilation and the level of ventilation is adjusted to maintain Pa_{CO_2} within tight limits.

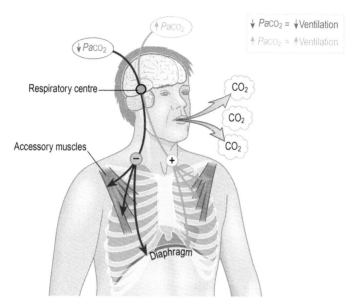

Figure 2 *Control of ventilation.*

A note on ... hypoxic drive

In patients with chronically high $PaCO_2$ levels (chronic hypercapnia), the specialised receptors that detect CO_2 levels can become desensitised. The body then relies on receptors that detect the PaO_2 to gauge the adequacy of ventilation and low PaO_2 becomes the principal ventilatory stimulus. This is referred to as *hypoxic drive*.

In patients who rely on hypoxic drive, overzealous correction of hypoxaemia, with supplemental O_2, may depress ventilation, leading to a catastrophic rise in $PaCO_2$. Patients with chronic hypercapnia must therefore be given supplemental O_2 in a controlled fashion with careful ABG monitoring. The same does not apply to patients with acute hypercapnia.

HAEMOGLOBIN OXYGEN SATURATION (SO_2)

Oxygenation is more complicated than CO_2 elimination. The first thing to realise is that the PO_2 does not actually tell us how much O_2 is in blood. It only measures free, unbound O_2 molecules – a tiny proportion of the total.

In fact, almost all O_2 molecules in blood are bound to a protein called *haemoglobin* (Hb; Figure 3). Because of this, the amount of O_2 in blood depends on the following two factors:

1. **Hb concentration:** This factor determines how much O_2 blood has *the capacity to carry.*

2. **Saturation of Hb with O_2 (SO_2):** This factor is the percentage of available binding sites on Hb that contain an O_2 molecule – i.e. *how much of the carrying capacity is being used* (Figure 4).

Note

$SO_2 = O_2$ saturation in (any) blood
$SaO_2 = O_2$ saturation in *arterial blood*

A note on ... pulse oximetry

SaO_2 can be measured using a probe (pulse oximeter) applied to the finger or earlobe. In most cases it provides adequate information to gauge oxygenation, but it is less accurate with saturations below 75% and unreliable when peripheral perfusion is poor. Oximetry does not provide information on $PaCO_2$ and, therefore, should not be used as a substitute for ABG analysis in ventilatory impairment.

Key point

PO_2 is not a measure of the amount of O_2 in blood – ultimately, the SaO_2 and the Hb concentration determine the O_2 content of arterial blood.

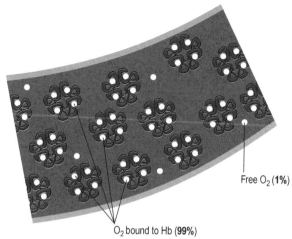

Free O_2 (**1%**)

O_2 bound to Hb (**99%**)

Figure 3 *Relative proportions of free O_2 molecules and O_2 molecules bound to haemoglobin in blood.*

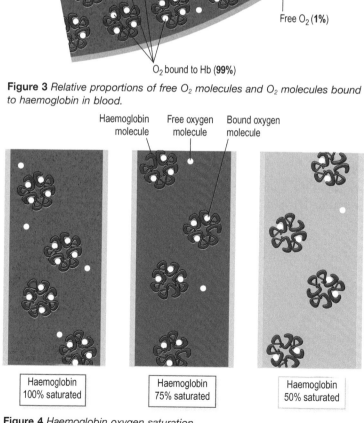

Haemoglobin molecule   Free oxygen molecule   Bound oxygen molecule

| Haemoglobin 100% saturated | Haemoglobin 75% saturated | Haemoglobin 50% saturated |

Figure 4 *Haemoglobin oxygen saturation.*

OXYHAEMOGLOBIN DISSOCIATION CURVE

We now know that the amount of O_2 in blood depends on the Hb concentration and the So_2. So what is the significance of the Po_2?

Po_2 can be thought of as the driving force for O_2 molecules to bind to Hb: as such, it regulates the So_2. The oxyhaemoglobin dissociation curve (Figure 5) shows the So_2 that will result from any given Po_2.

In general, the higher the Po_2, the higher the So_2, but *the curve is not linear*. The green line is known as the 'flat part of the curve': changes in Po_2 over this range have relatively little effect on the So_2. By contrast, the red line is known as the 'steep part of the curve': even small changes in Po_2 over this range may have a major impact on So_2.

Note that, with a 'normal' Pao_2 of approximately 13 kPa (100 mmHg), Hb is, more or less, *maximally saturated* ($Sao_2 > 95\%$). This means blood has used up its O_2-carrying capacity and any further increase in Pao_2 will *not* significantly increase arterial O_2 content.

Key point

Po_2 is not the amount of O_2 in blood but is the driving force for saturating Hb with O_2.

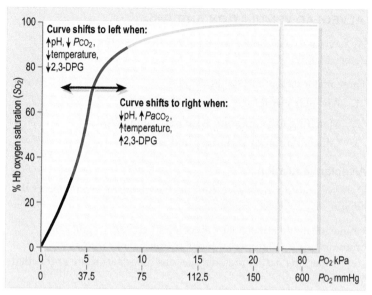

Figure 5 *Oxyhaemoglobin dissociation curve. The curve defines the relationship between Po_2 and the percentage saturation of haemoglobin with oxygen (So_2). Note the sigmoid shape: it is relatively flat when Po_2 is greater than 80 mmHg (10.6 kPa) but steep when Po_2 falls below 60 mmHg (8 kPa). 2,3-DPG = 2,3-diphosphoglycerate.*

Key point

When Hb approaches maximal O_2 saturation, further increases in Po_2 do not significantly increase blood O_2 content.

ALVEOLAR VENTILATION AND Pa_{O_2}

We have now seen how Pa_{O_2} regulates the Sa_{O_2}. But what determines Pa_{O_2}?

Three major factors dictate the Pa_{O_2}:

1. **Alveolar ventilation**
2. **Matching of ventilation with perfusion ($\dot{V}/\dot{Q}$)**
3. **Concentration of O_2 in inspired air (Fi_{O_2})**

Alveolar ventilation

O_2 moves rapidly from alveoli to the bloodstream – so *the higher the alveolar P_{O_2}, the higher the Pa_{O_2}.*

Unlike air in the atmosphere, alveolar air contains significant amounts of CO_2 (Figure 6). More CO_2 means a lower P_{O_2} (remember: the partial pressure of a gas reflects its share of the total volume).

An increase in alveolar ventilation allows more CO_2 to be 'blown off', resulting in a higher alveolar P_{O_2}. If, by contrast, ventilation declines, CO_2 accumulates at the expense of O_2 and alveolar P_{O_2} falls.

Whereas hyperventilation can increase alveolar P_{O_2} only slightly (bringing it closer to the P_{O_2} of inspired air), there is no limit to how far alveolar P_{O_2} (and hence Pa_{O_2}) can fall with inadequate ventilation.

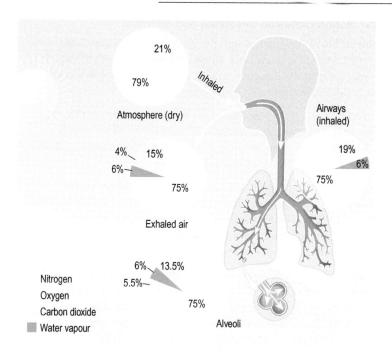

Figure 6 *Composition of inhaled and exhaled gases at various stages of respiration.*

Key point

Both oxygenation and CO_2 elimination depend on alveolar ventilation: impaired ventilation causes PaO_2 to fall and $PaCO_2$ to rise.

Ventilation/perfusion mismatch and shunting

Not all blood flowing through the lung meets well-ventilated alveoli and not all ventilated alveoli are perfused with blood – especially in the presence of lung disease. This problem is known as *ventilation/perfusion ($\dot{V}/\dot{Q}$) mismatch*.

Imagine if alveoli in one area of the lung are poorly ventilated (e.g. due to collapse or consolidation). Blood passing these alveoli returns to the arterial circulation with less O_2 and more CO_2 than normal. This is known as *shunting*[1] (Figure 7).

Now, by *hyperventilating*, we can shift more air in and out of our remaining 'good alveoli'. This allows them to blow-off extra CO_2 so that the blood passing them can offload more CO_2. The lower CO_2 in non-shunted blood compensates for the higher CO_2 in shunted blood, maintaining the $Pa{\scriptstyle CO_2}$.

The same does *NOT* apply to oxygenation. Blood passing 'good alveoli' is not able to carry more O_2 because its Hb is already maximally saturated with O_2 (remember: flat part of the curve, Figure 5). The non-shunted blood therefore cannot compensate for the low O_2 levels in shunted blood and the $Pa{\scriptstyle O_2}$ falls.

Key points

$\dot{V}/\dot{Q}$ mismatch allows poorly oxygenated blood to re-enter the arterial circulation, thus lowering $Pa{\scriptstyle O_2}$ and $Sa{\scriptstyle O_2}$.

Provided overall alveolar ventilation is maintained, the $\dot{V}/\dot{Q}$ mismatch does not lead to an increase in $Pa{\scriptstyle CO_2}$.

[1] *The term also applies to blood that bypasses alveoli altogether (anatomical shunting).*

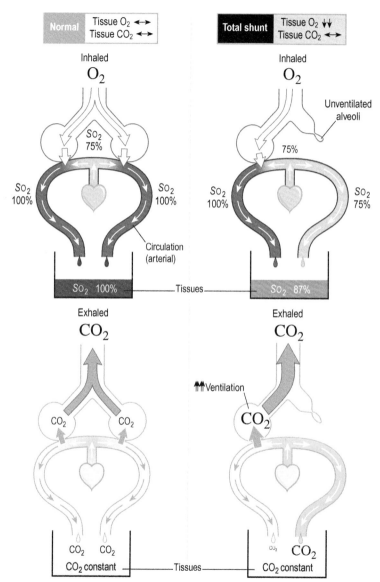

Figure 7 *Effect of shunt on oxygen and carbon dioxide.*

Fio_2 and oxygenation

The fraction of inspired oxygen (Fio_2) refers to the percentage of O_2 in the air we breathe in. The Fio_2 in room air is 21%, but can be increased with supplemental O_2.

A low Pao_2 may result from either $\dot{V}/\dot{Q}$ mismatch or inadequate ventilation and, in both cases, increasing the Fio_2 will improve the Pao_2. The exact Fio_2 requirement varies depending on how severely oxygenation is impaired and will help to determine the choice of delivery device (Figure 8). When the cause is inadequate ventilation, it must be remembered that increasing Fio_2 will not reverse the rise in $Paco_2$.

Supplemental O_2 makes ABG analysis more complex as it can be difficult to judge whether the Pao_2 is appropriately high for the Fio_2 and, hence, whether oxygenation is impaired. A useful rule of thumb is that the difference between Fio_2 and Pao_2 (in kPa) should not normally be greater than 10. However, there is often a degree of uncertainty regarding the precise Fio_2 and, if subtle impairment is suspected, the ABG should be repeated on room air.

Oxygen delivery devices

Nasal prongs: Fio_2 < 40%. Comfortable and convenient. Fio_2 non-specific: depends on flow rate (1–6 L/min) and ventilation.

Standard face mask: Fio_2 30–50% at flow rates 6–10 L/min but imprecise. May cause CO_2 retention at flows less than 5 L/min (rebreathing) and, therefore, not useful for providing lower Fio_2.

Fixed performance (high-flow) face mask: Fio_2 24–60%. Delivers fixed, predictable Fio_2. Ideal for providing controlled, accurate O_2 therapy at low concentrations.

Face mask with reservoir: Fio_2 60–80%. Can achieve even higher Fio_2 with a tight-fitting mask. Useful for short-term use in respiratory emergencies.

Endotracheal intubation: Fio_2 21–100%. Used in severely unwell patients with very high O_2 requirements, especially in patients with ventilatory failure. The patient is sedated and mechanically ventilated.

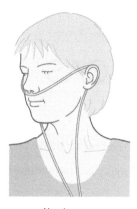

Nasal prongs

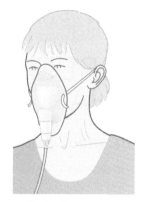

Fixed performance mask

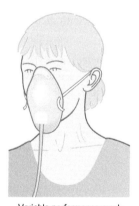

Variable performance mask

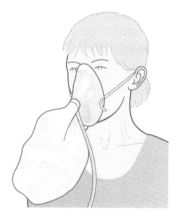

Mask with reservoir

Figure 8 *Oxygen delivery devices.*

DISORDERS OF GAS EXCHANGE

HYPOXIA, HYPOXAEMIA AND IMPAIRED OXYGENATION

The above terms are often used interchangeably but mean different things.

Hypoxia refers to *any state in which tissues receive an inadequate supply of O_2 to support normal aerobic metabolism*[1] (Figure 9). It may result from either hypoxaemia (see below) or impaired blood supply to tissues (ischaemia). It is often associated with lactic acidosis as cells resort to anaerobic metabolism.

Hypoxaemia refers to *any state in which the O_2 content of arterial blood is reduced*. It may result from impaired oxygenation (see below), low haemoglobin (anaemia) or reduced affinity of haemoglobin for O_2 (e.g. carbon monoxide).

Impaired oxygenation refers to *hypoxaemia resulting from reduced transfer of O_2 from lungs to the bloodstream*. It is identified by a low Pa_{O_2} (<10.7 kPa; <80 mmHg).

It is important to note the distinction between *impaired* oxygenation (which results in hypoxaemia) and *inadequate* oxygenation (which results in hypoxia). Consider a patient with a Pa_{O_2} of 8.5 kPa. The patient has impaired oxygenation, suggesting the presence of important lung disease. Nevertheless, the patient's Pa_{O_2} would usually result in an Sa_{O_2} greater than 90% and, *provided the haemoglobin and cardiac output are normal*, adequate O_2 delivery to tissues.

---

[1] *It is often advisable to use the term* tissue hypoxia *to avoid any confusion.*

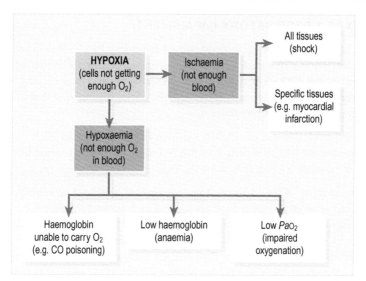

Figure 9 *Causes of hypoxia.*

TYPE 1 RESPIRATORY IMPAIRMENT

Type 1 respiratory impairment[2] is defined as low Pao_2 with normal or low $Paco_2$. This implies defective oxygenation despite adequate ventilation. $\dot{V}/\dot{Q}$ mismatch is usually responsible and may result from a number of causes (Box 1.3.1). The $Paco_2$ is often low due to compensatory hyperventilation.

If the arterial blood gas (ABG) is drawn from a patient on supplemental O_2, the Pao_2 may not be below the normal range, but will be inappropriately low for the Fio_2.

The severity of type 1 respiratory impairment is judged according to the scale of the resulting hypoxaemia and, ultimately, the presence of hypoxia (Table 1.3.1). Here it is important to remember the O_2 dissociation curve. Reductions in Pao_2 as far as 8 kPa have a relatively minor effect on Sao_2 and are well tolerated. Beyond this threshold, we reach the 'steep part' of the curve and further reductions in Pao_2 will lead to much greater falls in Sao_2, significantly lowering the O_2 content of arterial blood.

Initial treatment of type 1 respiratory impairment is aimed at achieving an adequate Pao_2 and Sao_2 with supplemental O_2 while attempting to correct the underlying cause. In many cases pulse oximetry can be used as an alternative to repeated ABG sampling to monitor progress.

[2]We use the term impairment *rather than* failure *here as the diagnosis of respiratory failure requires a Pao_2 less than 8 kPa (<60 mmHg).*

Box 1.3.1   Common causes of type 1 respiratory impairment*

Pneumonia	Acute asthma
Pulmonary embolism	Acute respiratory distress syndrome
Pneumothorax	Fibrosing alveolitis
Pulmonary oedema	Chronic obstructive pulmonary disease

*The usual mechanism is $\dot{V}/\dot{Q}$ mismatch; however, some conditions (e.g. alveolitis) impair diffusion of gases across the alveolar capillary membrane.

Table 1.3.1   Assessing severity of type 1 respiratory impairment

	Mild	Moderate	Severe
Pao_2 (kPa)	8–10.6	5.3–7.9	<5.3
Pao_2 (mmHg)	60–79	40–59	<40
Sao_2 (%)	90–94	75–89	<75

Other markers of severe impairment

- High Fio_2 requirements to maintain adequate Pao_2
- Lactic acidosis (indicating tissue hypoxia)
- Organ dysfunction (drowsiness, confusion, renal failure, haemodynamic collapse, coma)

TYPE 2 RESPIRATORY IMPAIRMENT

Type 2 respiratory impairment is defined by a high Pa_{CO_2} (hypercapnia) and is due to inadequate alveolar ventilation. Because oxygenation also depends on ventilation, the Pa_{O_2} is usually low, but may be normal if the patient is on supplemental O_2. It is important to note that any cause of type 1 impairment may lead to type 2 impairment if exhaustion supervenes (Box 1.3.2).

Acute rises in Pa_{CO_2} lead to dangerous accumulation of acid in the blood (see Section 1.4) and must be reversed. Chronic hypercapnia is accompanied by a rise in bicarbonate (HCO_3) level, which preserves acid–base balance. However, patients with chronic type 2 impairment who experience a further sharp decline in ventilation will also have a rapid rise in Pa_{CO_2} (acute on chronic), leading to acid accumulation and low blood pH (Table 1.3.2; Box 1.3.3).

Supplemental O_2 improves hypoxaemia but not hypercapnia and, therefore, treatment of type 2 respiratory impairment should also include measures to improve ventilation (e.g. reversal of sedation, relief of airways obstruction, assisted ventilation). The overzealous administration of supplemental O_2 to some patients with *chronic* type 2 impairment may further depress ventilation by abolishing hypoxic drive (p. 7).

Because pulse oximetry provides no information on Pa_{CO_2}, it is not a suitable substitute for ABG monitoring in type 2 respiratory impairment.

Table 1.3.2   The ABG in different patterns of type 2 impairment

	$Paco_2$	HCO_3	pH
Acute	↑	→	↓
Chronic	↑	↑	→
Acute on chronic	↑	↑	↓

Box 1.3.2   Common causes of type 2 respiratory impairment

Chronic obstructive pulmonary disease*   Opiate/benzodiazepine toxicity

Exhaustion   Inhaled foreign body

Flail chest injury   Neuromuscular disorders

Kyphoscoliosis   Obstructive sleep apnoea

*May lead to either type 1 or type 2 respiratory impairment.

Box 1.3.3   Clinical signs of hypercapnia

Confusion   Drowsiness

Flapping tremor   Bounding pulse

Warm extremities   Headache

HYPERVENTILATION

Hyperventilation leads to a low Pa_{CO_2} (hypocapnia) and a corresponding rise in blood pH (see Section 1.4). In chronic cases it is accompanied by a rise in HCO_3, which corrects blood pH. An increase in the rate and depth of breathing is usually apparent. A large drop in Pa_{CO_2} may lead to tingling around the mouth and extremities, light-headedness and even syncope.

Psychogenic hyperventilation often presents in a dramatic fashion, with patients complaining of severe breathlessness and an inability to take in enough air. It may be difficult to distinguish from respiratory disease. The ABG shows a low Pa_{CO_2} with a normal Pa_{O_2}.

Hyperventilation also occurs as a compensatory response to metabolic acidosis (secondary hyperventilation), as described in Section 1.4. Other causes are presented in Table 1.3.3.

Table 1.3.3	Common causes of hyperventilation	
Primary	Anxiety (psychogenic)	Pain or distress
	Hypoxaemia	Fever
	Salicylate toxicity	Central nervous system disorders
	Hepatic cirrhosis	
Secondary	Metabolic acidosis (of any aetiology)	

SUMMARY OF GAS EXCHANGE ABNORMALITIES

The four main patterns of ABG abnormality in disorders of gas exchange are summarised in Table 1.3.4.

Table 1.3.4 Patterns of ABG abnormality in disorders of gas exchange			
	Pao_2	$Paco_2$	HCO_3
Respiratory impairment			
Type 1	↓	↓/→	→
Acute type 2	↓/→	↑	→
Chronic type 2*	↓/→	↑	↑
Hyperventilation	→	↓	→/↓

*Acute on chronic distinguished from chronic by presence of ↑ H^+.

A note on ... the A – a gradient

The A – a gradient is the difference between the alveolar Po_2 (averaged across all alveoli) and the Po_2 in arterial blood. It tells us whether the Pao_2 is appropriate for the level of alveolar ventilation and is therefore a measure of the degree of $\dot{V}/\dot{Q}$ mismatch.

In practice, its main uses lie in detecting subtle increases in $\dot{V}/\dot{Q}$ mismatch where the Pao_2 is still within the normal range (e.g. pulmonary embolism) and identifying the presence of $\dot{V}/\dot{Q}$ mismatch in patients with type 2 respiratory impairment (this distinguishes pure type 2 respiratory impairment from mixed type 1 and type 2 impairment).

Calculation of the A – a gradient is not required for the scenarios in Part 2 of the book but, for those interested, a guide can be found in the Appendix.

ACID–BASE BALANCE: THE BASICS

The terms *acidity* and *alkalinity* simply refer to the concentration of free hydrogen ions (H^+) in a solution. H^+ concentration can be expressed directly in nanomoles per litre (nmol/L) or as pH (see facing page).

Solutions with high H^+ (low pH) are acidic and those with low H^+ (high pH) are alkaline. The point at which a substance changes from alkali to acid is the neutral point (pH = 7, H^+ = 100 nmol/L).

An *acid* is a substance that *releases* H^+ when it is dissolved in solution. Acids therefore increase the H^+ concentration of the solution (i.e. lower the pH). A *base* is a substance that *accepts* H^+ when dissolved in solution. Bases therefore lower the H^+ concentration of a solution (i.e. raise the pH). A *buffer* is a substance that can either accept or release H^+ depending on the surrounding H^+ concentration. Buffers therefore resist big changes in H^+ concentration.

Human blood normally has a pH of 7.35–7.45 (H^+ = 35–45 nmol/L) and, therefore, it is slightly alkaline. If blood pH is below the normal range (<7.35), there is an acidaemia. If it is above the normal range (>7.45), there is an alkalaemia.

An acidosis is any process that lowers blood pH, whereas an alkalosis is any process that raises blood pH.

What is pH?

The pH (power of hydrogen) scale is a simplified way of expressing large changes in H^+ concentration, though if you have not come across it before you might think it was designed just to confuse you!

It is a *negative logarithmic* scale (Figure 10). The 'negative' means that pH values get lower as the H^+ concentration increases (so a pH of 7.1 is more acidic than 7.2). The 'logarithmic' means that a shift in pH by one number represents a 10-fold change in H^+ concentration (so 7 is *10 times* more acidic than 8).

Why is acid–base balance important?

For cellular processes to occur efficiently, the H^+ concentration must be maintained within tight limits. Failure to maintain pH balance leads to inefficient cellular reactions and ultimately death (Figure 10).

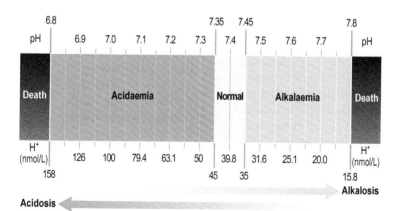

Figure 10 *pH/H^+ scale.*

MAINTAINING ACID–BASE BALANCE

What generates H⁺ ions in our bodies?

The breakdown of fats and sugars for energy generates CO_2, which, when dissolved in blood, forms carbonic acid (see Box on facing page).

Metabolism of protein produces hydrochloric acid, sulphuric acid and other so-called metabolic acids.

H^+ ions must, therefore, be removed to maintain normal blood pH.

What removes H⁺ ions from our bodies?

Respiratory mechanisms

Our lungs are responsible for removing CO_2. Pa_{CO_2}, the partial pressure of carbon dioxide in our blood, is determined by alveolar ventilation. If CO_2 production is altered, we adjust our breathing to exhale more or less CO_2, as necessary, to maintain Pa_{CO_2} within normal limits. The bulk of the acid produced by our bodies is in the form of CO_2, so it is our lungs that excrete the vast majority of the acid load.

Renal (metabolic) mechanisms

The kidneys are responsible for excreting metabolic acids. They secrete H^+ ions into urine and reabsorb HCO_3^- from urine. HCO_3^- is a base (and therefore accepts H^+ ions), so it reduces the concentration of H^+ ions in blood. The kidneys can adjust urinary H^+ and HCO_3^- excretion in response to changes in metabolic acid production. However, the kidneys do not just regulate acid–base balance; they must also maintain stable concentrations of the major electrolytes (e.g. sodium and potassium) and try to preserve *electroneutrality* (i.e. the overall balance between positively and negatively charged particles in the body). The need to perform these other tasks can sometimes interfere with pH regulation – either driving disturbances of acid–base balance or preventing their correction.

MAINTAINING ACID–BASE BALANCE

Just one equation...

The following equation is crucial to understanding acid–base balance:

$$H_2O + CO_2 \leftrightarrow H_2CO_3 \leftrightarrow H^+ + HCO_3^-$$

First, this equation shows that CO_2, when dissolved in blood, becomes an acid.

The more CO_2 added to blood, the more H_2CO_3 (carbonic acid) is produced, which dissociates to release free H^+.

Second, it predicts that blood pH depends not on the absolute amounts of CO_2 or HCO_3 present but on *the ratio of CO_2 to HCO_3*. Thus, a change in CO_2 will not lead to a change in pH if it is balanced by a change in HCO_3 that preserves the ratio (and vice versa). Because CO_2 is controlled by respiration and HCO_3 by renal excretion, this explains how compensation can prevent changes in blood pH.

Balancing acts in the kidney

There are two major 'balancing acts' that influence acid–base regulation:

1. Sodium ions (Na^+) are retained by swapping them for either a potassium ion (K^+) or H^+. When K^+ is in short supply, H^+ has to take up the slack (and vice versa), and therefore, more H^+ are excreted in exchange for Na^+.

2. Cl^- and HCO_3^- are the main negatively charged ions (anions) that have to balance with positively charged ions (cations; predominantly Na^+ and K^+). During times of high Cl^- loss, more HCO_3^- is retained; when HCO_3^- losses are high (via the kidney or gastrointestinal tract), more Cl^- is retained.

Therefore, generally speaking, K^+ and H^+ levels have a tendency to move in the same direction, whereas a primary fall in either Cl^- or HCO_3^- will usually cause the other to move in the opposite direction.

DISTURBANCES OF ACID–BASE BALANCE

An acidosis is any process that acts to lower blood pH. If it is due to a rise in Pa_{CO_2}, it is called a *respiratory acidosis*; if it is due to any other cause, then HCO_3 is reduced and it is called a *metabolic acidosis*.

An alkalosis is any process that acts to increase blood pH. If it is due to a fall in Pa_{CO_2}, it is called a *respiratory alkalosis*; if it is due to any other cause, then HCO_3 is raised and it is called a *metabolic alkalosis*.

Pa_{CO_2} raised = Respiratory acidosis
Pa_{CO_2} low = Respiratory alkalosis
HCO_3 raised = Metabolic alkalosis
HCO_3 low = Metabolic acidosis

The renal and respiratory systems operate jointly to maintain blood pH within normal limits. If one system is overwhelmed, leading to a change in blood pH, the other usually adjusts, automatically, to limit the disturbance (e.g. if kidneys fail to excrete metabolic acids, ventilation is increased to exhale more CO_2). This is known as *compensation*.

Acid–base disturbances can therefore be considered as a set of scales.

Normal acid–base balance

When acid–base balance is entirely normal, with no alkalotic or acidotic pressures, it is like having a set of scales with no weights on it (Figure 11).

Uncompensated acid–base disturbance

When an acidosis or alkalosis develops, the scales become unbalanced, leading to acidaemia or alkalaemia, respectively. In Figure 12, there is a primary respiratory acidosis with no opposing metabolic process.

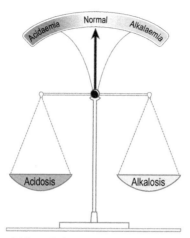

Figure 11 *Normal acid–base balance.*

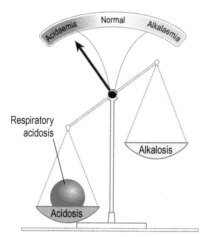

Figure 12 *Uncompensated respiratory acidosis.*

COMPENSATED ACID–BASE DISTURBANCE

As described earlier, a respiratory or metabolic disturbance is often *compensated* for by adjustment of the other system to offset the primary disturbance. Importantly, compensatory changes in respiration happen over minutes to hours, whereas metabolic responses take days to develop.

Figures 13 and 14 represent two scenarios in which the lungs have responded to a primary metabolic acidosis by increasing alveolar ventilation to eliminate more CO_2 (compensatory respiratory alkalosis). In Figure 13, an acidaemia persists despite compensation (partial compensation); in Figure 14, blood pH has returned to the normal range (full compensation).

When faced with such an ABG, how can we tell which is the primary disturbance and which is the compensatory process?

The first rule to remember is that *overcompensation does not occur*. The midpoint of the acid–base scales lies at a pH of 7.4 (H^+ 40). If the scales tip towards acidaemia (pH < 7.4), this suggests a primary acidotic process; if they tip towards alkalaemia (pH > 7.4), a primary alkalotic process is likely.

The second rule is that *the patient is more important than the ABG*. When considering an ABG, one must always take account of the clinical context. For example, if the patient in Figure 14 were a diabetic, with high levels of ketones in the urine, it would be obvious that the metabolic acidosis was a primary process (diabetic ketoacidosis).

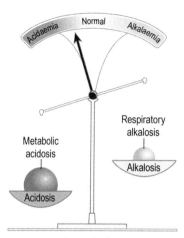

Figure 13 *Partially compensated metabolic acidosis.*

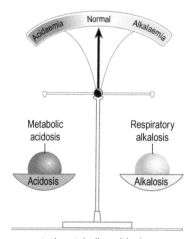

Figure 14 *Fully compensated metabolic acidosis.*

MIXED ACID–BASE DISTURBANCE

When a primary respiratory disturbance and primary metabolic disturbance occur simultaneously, there is said to be a *mixed* acid–base disturbance.

If these two processes oppose each other, the pattern will be similar to a compensated acid–base disturbance (Figure 14) and the resulting pH derangement will be minimised. A good example is salicylate poisoning, where primary hyperventilation (respiratory alkalosis) and metabolic acidosis (salicylate is acidic) occur independently.

By contrast, if the two processes cause pH to move in the same direction (metabolic acidosis and respiratory acidosis *or* metabolic alkalosis and respiratory alkalosis), a profound acidaemia or alkalaemia may result (Figure 15).

The nomogram

An alternative way to analyse ABGs is to use the acid–base nomogram (Figure 16). By plotting the $Pa\text{co}_2$ and H^+/pH values on the ABG nomogram, most ABGs can be analysed. If the plotted point lies outside the designated areas, this implies a mixed disturbance.

A note on ... predicting compensatory responses

It is not always easy to distinguish two primary opposing processes from a compensated disturbance. A more precise method than that described earlier involves calculating the expected compensatory response for any given primary disturbance. However, these calculations are usually unnecessary and are *not* required for the case scenarios in Part 2.

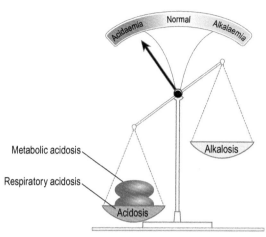

Figure 15 *Mixed respiratory and metabolic acidosis.*

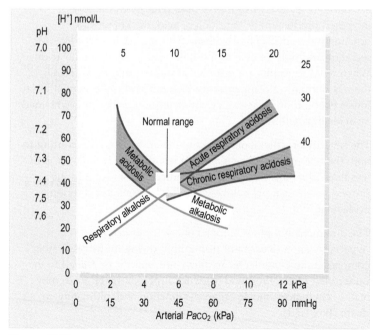

Figure 16 *The nomogram.*

DISORDERS OF ACID–BASE BALANCE

METABOLIC ACIDOSIS

A metabolic acidosis is any process, *other than a rise in* Pa_{CO_2}, that acts to lower blood pH. It is recognised on an ABG by a reduction in HCO_3 and a negative base excess (BE).

Metabolic acidosis may be caused by accumulation of metabolic acids (excess ingestion, increased production or reduced renal excretion) or by excessive loss of base (HCO_3). In the case of increased production or ingestion of acid, the kidneys (if functioning normally) have substantial capacity to boost H^+ secretion and may be able to forestall or, at least, attenuate acidosis. When renal measures are insufficient to prevent a fall in HCO_3, there is normally a compensatory increase in alveolar ventilation to lower Pa_{CO_2}. If this respiratory compensation is then overwhelmed, an acidaemia will result.

The severity of a metabolic acidosis should be judged according to both the underlying process and the resulting acidaemia. An HCO_3 less than 15 mmol/L (or BE < −10) indicates a severe acidotic process, whereas a pH below 7.25 (H^+ > 55) constitutes serious acidaemia.

The dominant symptom in metabolic acidosis is often hyperventilation (Kussmaul respiration) owing to the respiratory compensation. Other signs are fairly non-specific or related to the underlying cause. Profound acidaemia (pH < 7.15; H^+ > 70) may lead to circulatory shock, organ dysfunction and, ultimately, to death (Box 1.5.1).

Box 1.5.1   Metabolic acidosis (low HCO$_3$)

With raised anion gap

Lactic acidosis (e.g. hypoxaemia, ischaemia, shock, sepsis)
Ketoacidosis (diabetes, starvation, alcohol excess)
Renal failure (accumulation of sulphate, phosphate, urate)
Poisoning (aspirin, methanol, ethylene glycol)
Massive rhabdomyolysis

With normal anion gap

Renal tubular acidosis (types 1, 2 and 4)
Diarrhoea (HCO$_3^-$ loss)
Adrenal insufficiency
Ammonium chloride ingestion
Urinary diversion (e.g. ureterosigmoidostomy)
Drugs (e.g. acetazolamide)

METABOLIC ACIDOSIS AND THE ANION GAP

Calculating the anion gap (see facing page) may help to establish the cause of a metabolic acidosis.

Metabolic acidosis with a normal anion gap is usually caused by excessive loss of HCO_3^- through the renal tract (e.g. renal tubular acidosis) or the gastrointestinal tract (e.g. diarrhoea). The kidneys respond to the drop in HCO_3^- by retaining Cl^-, thereby preserving electroneutrality. Cl^- is one of the two measured anions in the equation on the facing page, and therefore, the anion gap remains normal. Because it entails an increase in Cl^-, normal anion gap acidosis is also referred to as 'hyperchloraemic metabolic acidosis'.

Metabolic acidosis with a high anion gap is usually caused by ingestion of an exogenous acid or increased production of an endogenous acid. Because the anion that is paired with H^+ to form these acids is typically not measured (e.g. lactate, salicylate), its presence leads to an increase in the gap. In high anion gap acidosis, the size of the gap is usually proportionate to the severity of the acidosis.

Lactic acidosis and diabetic ketoacidosis (DKA) – two common and clinically important causes of high anion gap metabolic acidosis – are discussed on the following pages. Other specific causes of metabolic acidosis are covered in the relevant cases in Part 2.

The anion gap explained

In blood, positively charged ions (cations) must be balanced by negatively charged ions (anions). However, when the two main cations ($Na^+ + K^+$) are compared with the two main anions ($Cl^- + HCO_3^-$), there appears to be a shortage of anions or an anion gap.

$$\text{Anion gap} = (Na^+ + K^+) - (Cl^- + HCO_3^-)$$

$$[\text{Normal} = 10\text{–}18 \text{ mmol/L}]$$

The gap is made up of unmeasured anions such as phosphate and sulphate and negatively charged proteins (these are difficult to measure).

A raised anion gap (>18 mmol/L) therefore indicates the presence of increased unmeasured anions.

Every acid consists of an H^+ ion paired with an anion. For example, lactic acid is the combination of H^+ with the negatively charged lactate ion. Thus, during conditions of increased lactic acid production there is accumulation of both H^+ (causing acidosis) and the lactate anion (causing a high anion gap).

LACTIC ACIDOSIS

This is the most common cause of metabolic acidosis in hospitalised patients. It is defined by a low HCO_3 in association with a plasma lactate concentration greater than 4 mmol/L (Figure 17).

When the supply of O_2 to tissues is inadequate to support normal aerobic metabolism, cells become dependent on anaerobic metabolism – a form of energy generation that does not require O_2 but generates lactic acid as a by-product. This can occur due to a problem with local blood supply (e.g. ischaemic gut or limb) or as a generalised failure of tissue oxygenation [e.g. profound hypoxaemia, shock (see below) or cardiac arrest]. The extent of lactic acidosis is an indicator of disease severity. In particular, the initial serum lactate concentration is a powerful predictor of death in patients with sepsis.

Rarely, lactic acidosis may, instead, be caused by drug toxicity (metformin), malignant tumours or mitochondrial dysfunction.

A note on 'shock'

Shock is a term used to denote a generalised failure of the circulation to provide adequate oxygenated blood to tissues. It is usually (but not always) associated with low blood pressure.

Inadequate perfusion of tissues can be detected through changes in skin (e.g. cold, mottled extremities) or organ dysfunction (e.g. reduced urine production) – but this is not always straightforward. By providing a 'global marker' of O_2 delivery to tissues, lactate levels can be very helpful in detecting the presence of shock and in monitoring response to treatment.

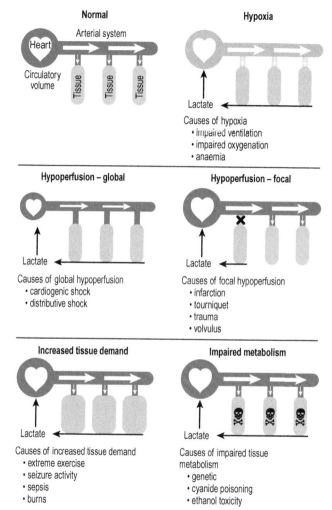

Figure 17 *Lactic acidosis.*

DIABETIC KETOACIDOSIS

DKA is a common and life-threatening form of metabolic acidosis caused by insulin deficiency. It tends to occur in patients with type 1 diabetes who are either presenting for the first time or have not been taking their usual insulin therapy. In the absence of insulin, the body cannot metabolise glucose and, therefore, increases metabolism of fats. The breakdown of fats produces ketones – small organic acids that provide an alternative source of energy but can accumulate, leading to acidosis. DKA is therefore characterised by the triad of:

1. **A high anion gap metabolic acidosis**
2. **An elevated plasma glucose (hyperglycaemia)**
3. **The presence of ketones (detectable in blood or urine)**

The severity of DKA is graded according to a variety of factors, including the severity of both the acidotic process and the resultant acidaemia (see Box 1.5.2). Patients are often profoundly dehydrated, with altered mental status.

In addition to respiratory compensation, increased urinary acid excretion (up to 30% of the total ketoacid load in patients with normal renal function) can serve to limit the acidaemia. Ketones can also be excreted as salts of sodium or potassium: that is, paired with Na^+ or K^+ rather than H^+. This lowers the anion gap without affecting the acidosis and helps to explain why patients develop a normal anion gap acidosis during treatment of DKA (another factor is intense Cl^- replacement in the form of intravenous normal saline).

OTHER FORMS OF KETOACIDOSIS

Not all ketoacidosis is caused by diabetes. Increased production of ketones can also occur in the setting of severe alcohol excess or starvation. In the former, there may be a profound acidosis, whereas ketoacidosis due to prolonged fasting is usually mild (e.g. $HCO_3 \geq$ 15 mmol/L). The absence of hyperglycaemia is often an important clue to these alternative causes.

Box 1.5.2 Diagnostic criteria and severity indicators for DKA

	Diagnostic criteria	Severe DKA
Acidosis*	pH < 7.3 or HCO_3 < 15 mmol/L	pH < 7.1 or HCO_3 < 5 mmol/L
Ketonaemia	>3 mmol/L (or >2+ on urine dip)	>6 mmol/L
Hyperglycaemia	>11 mmol/L (or known diabetes)	
Anion gap		>16 mmol/L
Other		GCS < 12; K < 3.5 mmol/L; SBP < 90 mmHg; HR > 100 or <60

Adapted from Joint British Diabetes Societies guideline: The Management of Diabetic Ketoacidosis in Adults, March 2010. http://www.diabetologists-abcd.org.uk/JBDS_DKA_Management.pdf.

*Guidelines specify that venous blood analysis is sufficiently accurate for measurement of pH and HCO_3 and an arterial sample is not required.

DKA, Diabetic ketoacidosis; *GCS*, Glasgow Coma Scale; *HR*, heart rate; *SBP*, systolic blood pressure.

METABOLIC ALKALOSIS

A metabolic alkalosis is any process, *other than a fall in* Pa_{CO_2}, that acts to increase blood pH. It is characterised on ABG by an elevated plasma HCO_3 and an increase in BE.

Respiratory compensation ($\uparrow Pa_{CO_2}$) occurs to limit the resulting alkalaemia but is limited by the need to avoid hypoxaemia. As a consequence, primary metabolic alkalosis is frequently accompanied by alkalaemia. By contrast, metabolic compensation for chronic respiratory acidosis (chronic type 2 respiratory failure) – a common cause of metabolic alkalosis in clinical practice – does not, by itself, result in alkalaemia.

Loss of H^+ ions may initiate the process (Box 1.5.3) but the kidneys have huge scope to correct threatened alkalosis by increasing HCO_3 excretion. Additional factors that impair this response are therefore also necessary. The usual suspects are depletion of chloride (Cl^-), potassium (K^+) and sodium (Na^+) ions – in most cases due to either sustained vomiting (Figure 18) or diuretic drugs. (See: 'Balancing acts in the kidney', p 29.)

Box 1.5.3 Metabolic alkalosis (high HCO₃)

Loss of gastric secretion (vomiting, NG suction)
Potassium depletion (e.g. diuretics)
Cushing syndrome
Conn syndrome (primary hyperaldosteronism)
Chloride-rich diarrhoea (e.g. villous adenoma)
Excessive administration of sodium bicarbonate

NG, nasogastric.

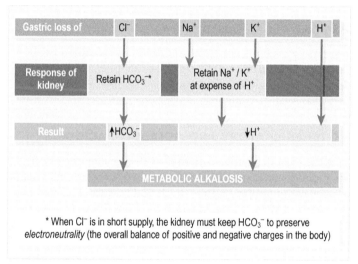

* When Cl⁻ is in short supply, the kidney must keep HCO₃⁻ to preserve
electroneutrality (the overall balance of positive and negative charges in the body)

Figure 18 *Effect of vomiting on acid–base balance.*

RESPIRATORY ACIDOSIS

A respiratory acidosis is, simply, *an increase in* Pa_{CO_2}. Because CO_2 dissolves in blood to form carbonic acid, this has the effect of lowering pH ($\uparrow H^+$ ions).

Normally, lungs are able to increase ventilation to maintain a normal Pa_{CO_2} – even in conditions of increased CO_2 production (e.g. sepsis). Thus, respiratory acidosis always implies a degree of reduced alveolar ventilation. This may occur from any cause of type 2 respiratory impairment (see Section 1.3) or to counteract a metabolic alkalosis.

RESPIRATORY ALKALOSIS

A respiratory alkalosis is *a decrease in* Pa_{CO_2} and is caused by alveolar hyperventilation. Primary causes are pain, anxiety (hyperventilation syndrome), fever, breathlessness and hypoxaemia. It may also occur to counteract a metabolic acidosis.

MIXED RESPIRATORY AND METABOLIC ACIDOSIS

This is the most dangerous pattern of acid–base abnormality. It leads to profound acidaemia as there are two simultaneous acidotic processes with no compensation. In clinical practice it is often due to severe ventilatory failure, in which the rising Pa_{CO_2} (respiratory acidosis) is accompanied by a low Pa_{O_2}, resulting in tissue hypoxia and consequent lactic acidosis.

Acute versus chronic respiratory acidosis

Because metabolic compensatory responses take days to develop, acute respiratory acidosis is almost always *uncompensated*, leading rapidly to profound and dangerous acidaemia. Indeed, an opposing metabolic alkalosis suggests that a respiratory acidosis must have been present for some time. In other words, the presence of metabolic compensation distinguishes chronic from acute type 2 ventilatory failure (see Section 1.3).

ABG SAMPLING TECHNIQUE

Before you can interpret an ABG you must, of course, obtain a sample of arterial blood. The following steps should be used as a guide (see also video on www.studentconsult.com) but the best way to learn is at the bedside with experienced supervision.

BEFORE SAMPLING

- Confirm the need for the ABG and identify any contraindications (Box 1.6.1).
- Always record details of O_2 therapy and respiratory support (e.g. ventilator settings).
- Unless results are required urgently, allow at least 20 minutes after any change in O_2 therapy before sampling (to achieve a steady state).
- Explain to the patient why you are doing the test, what it involves and the possible complications (bleeding, bruising, arterial thrombosis, infection and pain); then obtain consent to proceed.
- Prepare the necessary equipment (heparinised syringe with cap, 20–22G needle, sharps disposal container, gauze) and don universal precautions.
- Identify a suitable site for sampling by palpating the radial, brachial or femoral artery (Figure 19). Routine sampling should, initially, be attempted from the radial artery of the non-dominant arm.

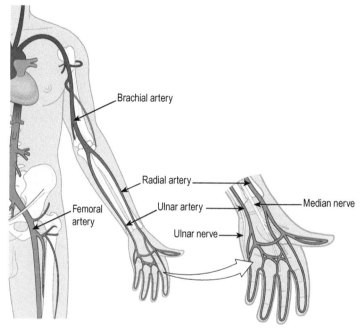

Figure 19 *Arterial puncture sites.*

Box 1.6.1 Contraindications to ABG analysis*

Inadequate collateral circulation at the puncture site

Should not be performed through a lesion or a surgical shunt

Evidence of peripheral vascular disease distant to the puncture site

A coagulopathy or medium- to high-dose anticoagulation therapy

*These are not absolute and depend on the clinical importance of ABG analysis.

RADIAL ARTERY SAMPLING

- Perform a modified Allen test to ensure adequate collateral circulation from the ulnar artery[1] (Figure 20).
- Position the patient's hand as shown in Figure 21, with the wrist extended 20–30 degrees. Greater extension of the wrist may impede arterial flow.
- Identify the radial artery by palpating the pulse; choose a site where the pulse is prominent.
- Clean the sampling site with an alcohol wipe.
- Expel the heparin from the syringe.
- Steady your hand on the patient's hand, as shown in Figure 21; then insert the needle at 45 degrees, bevel facing up.
- Be sure to insert the needle slowly to minimise the risk of arterial spasm.
- When the needle is in the artery, a flash of pulsatile blood will appear in the barrel of the needle. Most ABG syringes will then fill under arterial pressure (see info box on page 52).
- Obtain at least 3 mL of blood before withdrawing.

[1]However, the value of routinely performing a modified Allen test before arterial puncture has been questioned, in part due to its poor sensitivity and specificity for identifying inadequate collateral circulation (Slogoff S, Keats AS, Arlund C. On the safety of radial artery cannulation. Anaesthesiology 1983;59:42–47).

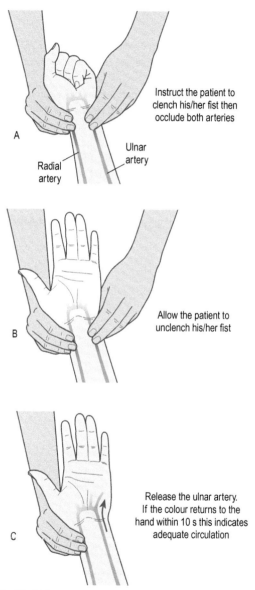

A — Instruct the patient to clench his/her fist then occlude both arteries

Ulnar artery

Radial artery

B — Allow the patient to unclench his/her fist

C — Release the ulnar artery. If the colour returns to the hand within 10 s this indicates adequate circulation

Figure 20 *Modified Allen test.*

AFTER SAMPLING

- Once adequate blood has been obtained, remove the needle and apply firm, direct pressure to the sample site for at least 5 minutes (and until bleeding has ceased).
- Dispose of all sharps and contaminated materials appropriately.
- Ensure no air bubbles are present in the sample, as they may compromise results. Any sample with more than very fine bubbles should be discarded.
- The sample should be analysed promptly: if the transit time is likely to exceed 10 minutes, then the syringe should be stored on crushed ice.
- If sampling is unsuccessful, it is often advisable to repeat the test on the opposite wrist as even slight irritation of the artery on the first attempt may have provoked arterial spasm, thwarting further attempts at puncture.

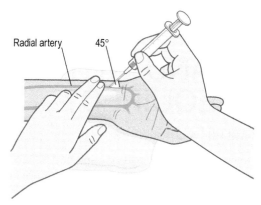
Radial artery   45°

Figure 21 *Positioning of the wrist for arterial blood gas sampling.*

Tip: local anaesthetic

Arterial sampling (particularly from the radial artery) can be extremely painful; discomfort can be reduced by injecting 1 mL of 1% lidocaine at the needle insertion site before sampling.

Venous or arterial blood?

Dark, non-pulsatile blood that requires manual suction to aspirate often indicates a venous sample (except in severe shock/cardiac arrest). Another clue is when SaO_2 on ABG analysis is significantly lower than SaO_2 on pulse oximetry.

WHEN AND WHY IS AN ABG REQUIRED?

1. TO ESTABLISH A DIAGNOSIS

The ABG is integral to the diagnosis of respiratory failure and primary hyperventilation. It also identifies the presence of metabolic acidosis and alkalosis. Other indications are listed in Box 1.7.1.

2. TO ASSESS ILLNESS SEVERITY

The four ABG values shown below, *in addition to overall clinical assessment*, may help identify critically unwell patients requiring urgent intervention.

$PaO_2 < 8$ kPa
Below 8 kPa, any fall in PaO_2 will produce a marked reduction in SaO_2 (the 'steep' part of the O_2 dissociation curve) and may lead to life-threatening hypoxaemia.
Rising $PaCO_2$
Because renal compensation occurs over days to weeks, acute rises in $PaCO_2$ produce a corresponding drop in pH. In respiratory distress, rising $PaCO_2$ often signifies exhaustion and is an ominous sign. Patients require urgent reversal of the process, leading to ventilatory failure or assisted ventilation.
BE < -10/$HCO_3 < 15$
This value is included in several severity scoring systems and, when due to lactic acidosis, indicates severe hypoxia at the cellular level.
$H^+ > 55$/pH < 7.25
A significant decrease in pH outside the normal range indicates that compensatory mechanisms have been overwhelmed and is a medical emergency.

3. TO GUIDE AND MONITOR TREATMENT

Regular ABG monitoring can help provide early warning of deterioration and judge the effectiveness of therapeutic interventions. It is essential for titrating O_2 therapy in patients with chronic type 2 respiratory failure and for optimising ventilator settings.

Box 1.7.1   Clinical scenarios in which an ABG is useful

Establishing diagnosis and assessing illness severity

Suspected hypercapnia ($\uparrow PaCO_2$)
  Drowsiness, flapping tremor, bounding pulses
  Clinical deterioration in a patient with chronic type 2 respiratory
  impairment or predisposing condition (e.g. chronic obstructive pulmonary
  disease)
Suspected severe hypoxaemia
  Very low or unrecordable O_2 saturation; cyanosis
Severe, prolonged or worsening respiratory distress
Smoke inhalation (carboxyhaemoglobin level)
Hyperventilation (confirm $\downarrow PaCO_2$, check for underlying metabolic acidosis)
Acute deterioration in consciousness
Any severely unwell patient*
Pulse oximetry unreliable or suspicious result
As part of a recognised illness severity scoring system (e.g. Glasgow
criteria in pancreatitis)

Guiding treatment and monitoring response

Mechanically ventilated patients
Patients receiving non-invasive assisted ventilation
Patients with respiratory failure
Patients with chronic hypercapnia receiving O_2
Critically ill patients undergoing surgery
Candidates for long-term oxygen therapy

*Including, but not restricted to, shock, sepsis, burns, major trauma, acute abdomen, poisoning, cardiac/renal/hepatic failure and diabetic ketoacidosis.

---

4. VENOUS BLOOD GAS ANALYSIS

Obtaining a venous blood sample is quicker, simpler and less painful than obtaining an arterial blood sample and avoids the potential complications of arterial puncture. Venous blood gas (VBG) analysis can yield clinically useful information and has become increasingly popular as an alternative to ABG in some clinical settings, especially within emergency departments. In some situations, analysis of venous blood can provide enough information to assist in clinical decisions; for example, VBG is now deemed adequate for both the diagnosis and the monitoring of diabetic ketoacidosis in the latest UK guidelines (Box 1.5.2; p. 43). However, it is also important to recognise the limitations of VBG in relation to arterial analysis. The following is therefore a rough guide to the use of VBG:

- There are large discrepancies between the P_{O_2} measured in arterial and venous blood. Therefore, VBG cannot be used to assess oxygenation.
- There is poor agreement between P_{CO_2} measured in venous and arterial blood. Although VBG values tend to be lower than ABG, the relationship is unpredictable. VBG should therefore not be used as a direct substitute for ABG in the measurement of P_{CO_2}. By contrast, a venous P_{CO_2} less than 45 mmHg makes significant arterial hypercapnia unlikely and, therefore, may avert the need for arterial puncture in some patients.
- There is good agreement between pH measured in venous and arterial blood. VBG may, therefore, be useful to screen for overall acid–base status. Based on limited data, there is also reasonably good agreement between VBG and ABG for HCO_3.
- In the setting of significant lactic acidosis, the actual lactate level may differ widely between ABG and VBG. However, a normal venous lactate level makes lactic acidosis unlikely.
- It is unclear whether the aforementioned relationships between ABG and VBG are preserved in the setting of shock or cardiac failure.
- Regional ischaemia caused by the use of a tourniquet has the potential to alter local acid–base metabolism; a tourniquet should, therefore, be released at least 1 minute before drawing blood for VBG or, preferably, avoided altogether.

COMMON ABG VALUES

The following parameters are commonly found on ABG reports and are provided for reference (normal ranges in parentheses):

H^+ (35–45 nmol/L) < 35 = alkalaemia,   > 45 = acidaemia

Concentration of free hydrogen ions (H^+): this is a measure of how acidic or alkaline a solution is.

pH (7.35–7.45) < 7.35 = acidaemia,   > 7.45 = alkalaemia

Negative log of the H^+ concentration: this is a common representation of the H^+ concentration. Because of the logarithmic nature of the scale, small changes in the pH actually represent large changes in the H^+ concentration.

Po_2 (> 10.6 kPa or > 80 mmHg in arterial blood on room air)

Partial pressure of O_2: can be thought of as the drive for O_2 molecules to move from one place to another. Po_2 is not a measure of O_2 content but it does determine the extent to which haemoglobin is saturated with O_2. Pao_2 refers *specifically* to the partial pressure of O_2 in *arterial blood*.

Pco_2 (4.7–6.0 kPa or 35–45 mmHg in arterial blood)

Partial pressure of CO_2: can be thought of as the drive for CO_2 molecules to move from one place to another and (unlike Po_2) is directly proportional to the amount of CO_2 in blood. $Paco_2$ refers *specifically* to the partial pressure of CO_2 in *arterial blood*.

So_2 (> 96% on room air)

O_2 saturation of haemoglobin: the percentage of O_2 binding sites on haemoglobin proteins occupied by O_2 molecules. This is a measure of how much of the blood's O_2-carrying capacity is being used. Sao_2 refers *specifically* to the O_2 saturation of *arterial blood*.

HCO$_3$act (22–28 mmol/L)

Actual bicarbonate: the plasma bicarbonate concentration *calculated from* the actual $P\text{co}_2$ and pH measurements in the arterial blood sample. High bicarbonate levels signify a metabolic alkalosis and low levels signify a metabolic acidosis.

HCO$_3$st (22–28 mmol/L)

Standard bicarbonate: the plasma bicarbonate concentration *calculated from* the $P\text{co}_2$ and pH measurements in the arterial blood sample after the $P\text{co}_2$ in the sample has been corrected to 5.3 kPa (40 mmHg). The authors recommend using this measurement of bicarbonate in ABG analysis.

BE (–2 to +2)

Base excess (BE): a calculation of the amount of base that needs to be added to, or removed from, a sample of blood to achieve a neutral pH, at 37°C, *after $P\text{co}_2$ has been corrected to 5.3 kPa (40 mmHg)*. A positive BE indicates that there is more base than normal (metabolic alkalosis) and a negative BE indicates that there is less base than normal (metabolic acidosis).

Lactate (0.4–1.5 mmol/L)

An indirect measure of lactic acid: high levels of lactic acid are usually a sign of tissue hypoxia.

Hb (13–18 g/dL for men, 11.5–16 g/dL for women)

Plasma haemoglobin concentration: this effectively determines the blood's capacity to carry O_2.

Na (135–145 mmol/L)

Plasma sodium concentration.

K (3.5–5 mmol/L)

Plasma potassium concentration.

Cl (95–105 mmol/L)

Plasma chloride concentration.

iCa (1.0–1.25 mmol/L)

Plasma ionised calcium concentration.

Glucose (3.5–5.5 mmol/L if fasting)

Plasma glucose concentration.

MAKING ABG INTERPRETATION EASY

The golden rule for making ABG interpretation easy is to assess pulmonary gas exchange and acid–base status *independently* (Figures 22 and 23).

ASSESSING PULMONARY GAS EXCHANGE

- Using the algorithm in Figure 22, classify gas exchange into one of the four possible categories.
- If there is type 1 respiratory impairment, assess severity of hypoxaemia (Table 1.9.1).
- If there is type 2 respiratory impairment, establish whether it is chronic or acute, then assess severity of hypercapnia and hypoxaemia (Table 1.9.1 and Box 1.9.1).
- If the category is hyperventilation, determine whether it is primary or secondary.

Table 1.9.1 Assessing hypoxaemia severity

	PaO_2	SaO_2
Mild	8–10.6 kPa 60–79 mmHg	90–94%
Moderate	5.3–7.9 kPa 40–59 mmHg	75–89%
Severe	<5.3 kPa <40 mmHg *or:* High FiO_2 requirements to maintain adequate PaO_2	<75%

Box 1.9.1 Assessing hypercapnia severity

Severity is not related to absolute $PaCO_2$ value but to the *rate of* $PaCO_2$ *rise* and degree of blood pH derangement (pH < 7.25 = severe acidaemia). The presence of exhaustion is also an ominous sign.

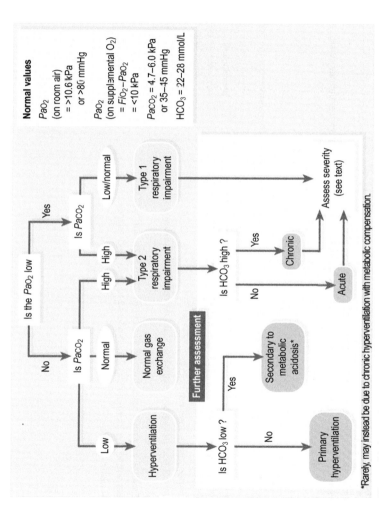

Normal values

PaO_2
(on room air)
= >10.6 kPa
or >80 mmHg

PaO_2
(on supplemental O_2)
= FiO_2–PaO_2
= <10 kPa

$PaCO_2$ = 4.7–6.0 kPa
or 35–45 mmHg

HCO_3 = 22–28 mmol/L

Is the PaO_2 low

No — Is $PaCO_2$

Yes — Is $PaCO_2$

Low → Hyperventilation

Normal → Normal gas exchange

High → Type 2 respiratory impairment

High → Type 2 respiratory impairment

Low/normal → Type 1 respiratory impairment

Further assessment

Is HCO_3 low ?

Yes → Secondary to metabolic acidosis*

No → Primary hyperventilation

Is HCO_3 high ?

Yes → Chronic → Assess severity (see text)

No → Acute → Assess severity (see text)

Type 1 respiratory impairment → Assess severity (see text)

*Rarely, may instead be due to chronic hyperventilation with metabolic compensation.

Figure 22 *Assessing pulmonary gas exchange.*

INTERPRETING ACID–BASE STATUS

- Use the flow chart in Figure 23 to broadly classify acid–base status.
- If the patient has a metabolic acidosis, calculate the anion gap to narrow down the differential diagnosis.

$$\text{Anion gap} = (Na^+ + K^+) - (Cl^- + HCO_3^-)$$

$$\text{Normal} = 10\text{–}18\,\text{mmol/L}$$

- If the precise acid–base derangement is not immediately clear (e.g. middle column), then remember the following points:
  - Always consider the clinical context when interpreting acid–base status.
  - Metabolic compensation takes days to occur, respiratory compensation takes minutes.
  - Overcompensation does not occur.
  - An apparent compensatory response could represent an opposing primary process.
- Note that with a very mild acidaemia or alkalaemia, both $P\text{CO}_2$ and HCO_3 may be just within the 'normal range' (considered to be a mild mixed acid–base disturbance).

Normal values

$Pa\text{CO}_2 = 4.7\text{–}6.0\,\text{kPa}$
or $35\text{–}45\,\text{mmHg}$

BE (-2 to $+2$)

HCO_3st ($22\text{–}28\,\text{mmol/L}$)

pH ($7.35\text{–}7.45$)

H^+ ($35\text{–}45\,\text{nmol/L}$)

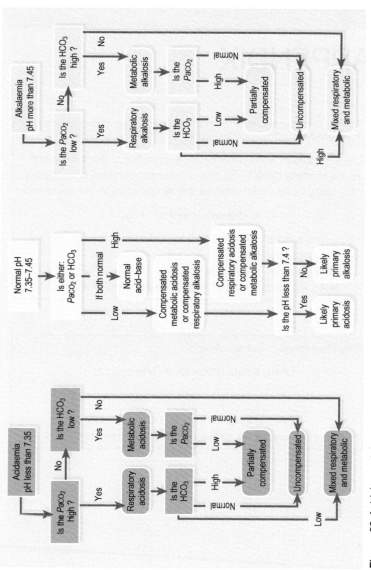

Figure 23 *Acid–base status.*

APPENDIX

A – a gradient

The A – a gradient is the difference between the Po_2 in alveoli (PAo_2) and the Po_2 in arterial blood (Pao_2). Pao_2 is measured on arterial blood gas but PAo_2 has to be calculated using the alveolar gas equation (see box below).

$$A – a\ gradient = PAo_2 – Pao_2$$

It is normally less than 2.6 kPa (20 mmHg), although it increases with age and Fio_2. This means that:

1. The normal range for Pao_2 falls with age
2. The A – a gradient is most accurate when performed on room air

Simplified alveolar gas equation*

$$PAo_2\ (kPa) = (Fio_2 \times 93.8) – (Paco_2 \times 1.2)$$

or

$$PAo_2\ (mmHg) = (Fio_2 \times 713) – (Paco_2 \times 1.2)$$

*Assumes the patient is at the sea level and has a body temperature of 37°C.

PART 2

THE ABG IN PRACTICE

CASES

History

A 25-year-old man, with no significant medical history, presents to the emergency department with a 2-day history of fever, productive cough and worsening breathlessness.

Examination

He is hot and flushed with a temperature of 39.3°C. He does not appear distressed but is using accessory muscles of respiration. There is diminished chest expansion on the left with dullness to percussion, bronchial breathing and coarse crackles in the left lower zone posteriorly.

Pulse	104 beats/min
Respiratory rate	28 breaths/min
Blood pressure	118/70 mmHg
Sao_2 (room air)	89%

Arterial blood gas 23 July 2014 Unit no.: 00654545 ID: John S.	**On room air**	
		Normal
H^+	31.8 nmol/L	(35–45)
pH	7.50	(7.35–7.45)
P_{CO_2}	3.74 kPa	(4.7–6.0)
	28.1 mmHg	(35–45)
P_{O_2}	7.68 kPa	(>10.6)
	57.8 mmHg	(>80)
Bicarb	23.9 mmol/L	(22–28)
BE	–0.5 mmol/L	(–2 to +2)
S_{O_2}	88.7%	(>96%)
Lactate	1.2 mmol/L	(0.4–1.5)
K	3.7 mmol/L	(3.5–5)
Na	138 mmol/L	(135–145)
Cl	99 mmol/L	(95–105)
iCa^+	1.2 mmol/L	(1–1.25)
Hb	15 g/dL	(13–18)
Glucose	5.4 mmol/L	(3.5–5.5)

Questions

1. a) Describe his gas exchange.
   b) Describe his acid–base status.
2. Should the patient receive supplemental O_2?
3. Is pulse oximetry a suitable alternative to repeated ABG monitoring in this case?

CASE 2

History

A 34-year-old morbidly obese woman with a body mass index of 49 has an ABG sample taken as part of her preoperative assessment for weight reduction surgery.

Apart from morbid obesity and type 2 diabetes, she is otherwise well and has no respiratory symptoms.

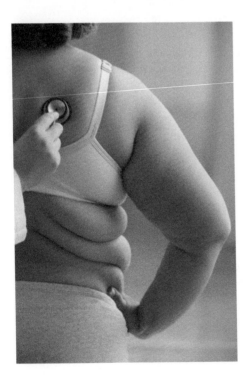

Arterial blood gas 14 Jan. 2014 Unit no.: 55392088 ID: Marcella P.	**On air**	
		Normal
H⁺	45 nmol/L	(35–45)
pH	7.35	(7.35–7.45)
P_{CO_2}	7.3 kPa	(4.7–6.0)
	54.8 mmHg	(35–45)
P_{O_2}	9.6 kPa	(>10.6)
	72.2 mmHg	(>80)
Bicarb	29 mmol/L	(22–28)
BE	+3.8 mmol/L	(–2 to +2)
S_{O_2}	96%	(>96%)
Lactate	1 mmol/L	(0.4–1.5)
K	4.7 mmol/L	(3.5–5)
Na	134 mmol/L	(135–145)
Cl	102 mmol/L	(95–105)
iCa⁺	1.2 mmol/L	(1–1.25)
Hb	13 g/dL	(11.5–16)
Glucose	9 mmol/L	(3.5–5.5)

Questions

1. a) Describe her gas exchange.
    b) Describe her acid–base status.
2. What is the most likely diagnosis?

CASE 3

History

A 24-year-old female nursing student attends hospital complaining of sudden-onset breathlessness. She flew to the UK from Australia the previous day and is very concerned she may have a pulmonary embolism. She has no pleuritic pain, haemoptysis or leg swelling, no history of lung disease or deep-vein thrombosis, and is a non-smoker.

Examination

She appears anxious and distressed. Her respiratory rate is elevated but chest examination is unremarkable and there are no clinical signs of deep-vein thrombosis. A chest X-ray reveals no abnormalities.

Pulse	88 beats/min
Respiratory rate	22 breaths/min
Blood pressure	124/76 mmHg
SaO_2 (room air)	95%

Arterial room gas
23 July 2014
Unit no.: 00654545
ID: Jill R.

On room air

		Normal
H^+	31.2 nmol/L	(35–45)
pH	7.51	(7.35–7.45)
P_{CO_2}	3.90 kPa	(4.7–6.0)
	29.3 mmHg	(35–45)
P_{O_2}	10.3 kPa	(>10.6)
	77.0 mmHg	(>80)
Bicarb	25.0 mmol/L	(22–28)
BE	+0.7 mmol/L	(−2 to +2)
S_{O_2}	93.7%	(>96%)
Lactate	1.0 mmol/L	(0.4–1.5)
K	4.3 mmol/L	(3.5–5)
Na	141 mmol/L	(135–145)
Cl	101 mmol/L	(95–105)
iCa^+	1.2 mmol/L	(1–1.25)
Hb	13 g/dL	(11.5–16)
Glucose	4.6 mmol/L	(3.5–5.5)

Questions

1. a) Describe her gas exchange.
   b) Describe her acid–base status.
2. What is the most likely diagnosis?

CASE 4

History

A 78-year-old man on a surgical ward is found unresponsive, having returned, a few hours before, from a complicated open cholecystectomy.

A review of his charts reveals that he has received three 10 mg injections of morphine since returning to the ward, in addition to the morphine delivered by his patient-controlled analgesia device.

Examination

The patient is unresponsive with shallow respirations and bilateral pinpoint pupils.

Pulse rate	90 beats/min
Respiratory rate	5 breaths/min
Blood pressure	98/64 mmHg
SaO_2	99%
BM (blood glucose)	5.6 mmol/L

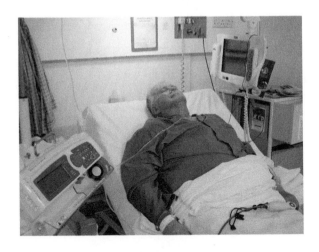

Arterial blood gas		**On 28% O$_2$**
18 Nov. 2013		
Unit no.: 6799986		
ID: Henry S.		
		Normal
H$^+$	65.4 nmol/L	(35–45)
pH	7.18	(7.35–7.45)
P$_{CO_2}$	8.2 kPa	(4.7–6.0)
	62 mmHg	(35–45)
P$_{O_2}$	11.76 kPa	(>10.6)
	87 mmHg	(>80)
Bicarb	22.4 mmol/L	(22–28)
BE	−1.5 mmol/L	(−2 to +2)
S$_{O_2}$	99.8%	(>96%)
Lactate	1 mmol/L	(0.4–1.5)
K	4.4 mmol/L	(3.5–5)
Na	137 mmol/L	(135–145)
Cl	103 mmol/L	(95–105)
iCa$^+$	1.16 mmol/L	(1–1.25)
Hb	11 g/dL	(13–18)
Glucose	3.9 mmol/L	(3.5–5.5)

Questions

1. a) Describe his gas exchange.
   b) Describe his acid–base status.
2. What is the most likely diagnosis?
3. What treatment does this patient require?

CASE 5

History

A 75-year-old man is brought into the emergency department by his family. He is extremely short of breath and struggling to speak.

Following a conversation with his family, it emerges that he has a long history of chronic obstructive pulmonary disease.

Over the last 3 days his breathing has worsened considerably and he has expectorated increased volumes of sputum.

Examination

The patient is struggling for breath and appears extremely distressed. He exhibits signs of chest hyperinflation and is breathing through pursed lips. Breath sounds are generally diminished but there are no added sounds.

Pulse	120 beats/min
Respiratory rate	26 breaths/min
Blood pressure	150/80 mmHg
Temperature	36°C
SaO_2%	81%

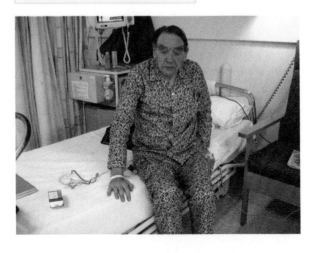

Arterial blood gas	**On air**	
10 Feb. 2014		
Unit no.: 77655349		
ID: Joseph S.		
		Normal
H^+	39.5 nmol/L	(35–45)
pH	7.40	(7.35–7.45)
P_{CO_2}	4.9 kPa	(4.7–6.0)
	36 mmHg	(35–45)
P_{O_2}	5.8 kPa	(>10.6)
	44 mmHg	(>80)
Bicarb	23 mmol/L	(22–28)
BE	–1.2 mmol/L	(–2 to +2)
S_{O_2}	80%	(>96%)
Lactate	1.0 mmol/L	(0.4–1.5)
K	4.1 mmol/L	(3.5–5)
Na	137 mmol/L	(135–145)
Cl	99 mmol/L	(95–105)
iCa^+	1.1 mmol/L	(1–1.25)
Hb	16.5 g/dL	(13–18)
Glucose	3.8 mmol/L	(3.5–5.5)

Questions

1. a) Describe his gas exchange.
   b) Describe his acid–base status.
2. Should you provide him with oxygen?

CASE 6

History

The patient from Case 5 is treated in the emergency department with nebulised bronchodilators, oral prednisolone and antibiotics. He is then transferred to a respiratory ward where he is administered 28% oxygen by a fixed concentration mask. Despite this, his Sao_2 (as measured by pulse oximetry) increases only marginally and there is no improvement in his symptoms.

Examination

Examination findings in the chest are unchanged but he now appears exhausted and slightly confused.

Pulse	120 beats/min
Respiratory rate	16 breaths/min
Blood pressure	120/80 mmHg
Sao_2	83% (on 28% O_2)
Temperature	36°C

A repeat ABG is performed (6 h after the first ABG).

Arterial blood gas		**On 28% O_2**
11 Feb. 2014		
Unit no.: 77655349		
ID: Joseph S.		
		Normal
H^+	51.4 nmol/L	(35–45)
pH	7.29	(7.35–7.45)
P_{CO_2}	6.9 kPa	(4.7–6.0)
	52 mmHg	(35–45)
P_{O_2}	6.4 kPa	(>10.6)
	48 mmHg	(>80)
Bicarb	24 mmol/L	(22–28)
BE	–0.9 mmol/L	(–2 to +2)
S_{O_2}	84%	(>96%)
Lactate	1.0 mmol/L	(0.4–1.5)
K	4.0 mmol/L	(3.5–5)
Na	137 mmol/L	(135–145)
Cl	99 mmol/L	(95–105)
iCa^+	1.1 mmol/L	(1–1.25)
Hb	16.5 g/dL	(13–18)
Glucose	4.2 mmol/L	(3.5–5.5)

Questions

1. a) Describe his gas exchange.
   b) Describe his acid–base status.
2. Should his oxygen now be stopped?

CASE 7

The patient from Cases 5 and 6 goes on to make a full recovery from his acute exacerbation. At outpatient review 3 months later, he remains dyspnoeic on mild exertion despite optimal therapy (including smoking cessation). His Sp_{O_2} on room air is noted to be 87%. He has no features to suggest acute exacerbation.

Arterial blood gas		**On air**
21 May 2014		
Unit no.: 77655349		
ID: Joseph S.		
		Normal
H^+	41 nmol/L	(35–45)
pH	7.42	(7.35–7.45)
P_{CO_2}	5.0 kPa	(4.7–6.0)
	mmHg	(35–45)
P_{O_2}	7.0 kPa	(>10.6)
	mmHg	(>80)
Bicarb	24 mmol/L	(22–28)
BE	–1.3 mmol/L	(–2 to +2)
S_{O_2}	87%	(>96%)
Lactate	1.1 mmol/L	(0.4–1.5)
K	4.1 mmol/L	(3.5–5)
Na	137 mmol/L	(135–145)
Cl	98 mmol/L	(95–105)
iCa^+	1.1 mmol/L	(1–1.25)
Hb	17.2 g/dL	(13–18)
Glucose	4.4 mmol/L	(3.5–5.5)

Questions

1. a) Describe his gas exchange.
   b) Describe his acid–base status.
2. What treatment should now be considered?

CASE 8

History

A 77-year-old woman is admitted to the stroke ward with right-sided weakness, visual disturbance and slurred speech. She is commenced on nasogastric feeding due to swallowing problems but has a large vomit 24 h later. She initially appears well but over the next few hours develops worsening breathing difficulties.

Examination

She is agitated, distressed and pyrexial. A dull percussion note and coarse crackles are evident at both lung bases. Other than acute confusion, neurological findings are unchanged from admission.

Pulse	92 beats/min
Respiratory rate	28 breaths/min
Blood pressure	112/65 mmHg
SaO_2 (60% O_2)	92%

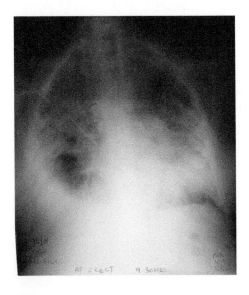

Arterial blood gas		**On 60% O$_2$**
23 July 2014		
Unit no.: 00654545		
ID: Mary W.		
		Normal
H$^+$	38.8 nmol/L	(35–45)
pH	7.41	(7.35–7.45)
P$_{CO_2}$	4.43 kPa	(4.7–6.0)
	33.2 mmHg	(35–45)
P$_{O_2}$	8.67 kPa	(>10.6)
	65.0 mmHg	(>80)
Bicarb	21.2 mmol/L	(22–28)
BE	−2.8 mmol/L	(−2 to +2)
S$_{O_2}$	92.7%	(>96%)
Lactate	1.6 mmol/L	(0.4–1.5)
K	4.0 mmol/L	(3.5–5)
Na	144 mmol/L	(135–145)
Cl	103 mmol/L	(95–105)
iCa$^+$	1.2 mmol/L	(1–1.25)
Hb	13 g/dL	(11.5–16)
Glucose	6.6 mmol/L	(3.5–5.5)

Questions

1. a) Describe her gas exchange.
   b) Describe her acid–base status.
2. What is the most likely diagnosis?
3. Is her condition mild, moderate or severe?

CASE 9

History

A 68-year-old man with chronic obstructive pulmonary disease is referred to hospital by his doctor with a short history of increased breathlessness and reduced effort tolerance. He is normally capable of walking around 500 m but now has difficulty dressing and is breathless at rest.

Examination

He is lucid, alert and mildly distressed. He is using accessory muscles of respiration and breathing through pursed lips. Chest examination reveals features of hyperinflation, generally diminished breath sounds and scattered rhonchi (wheeze).

Pulse	96 beats/min
Respiratory rate	24 breaths/min
Blood pressure	138/82 mmHg
SaO_2 (room air)	78%

Arterial blood gas	**On air**	
23 June 2014		
Unit no.: 00654545		
ID: Hamish R.		
		Normal
H^+	43.2 nmol/L	(35–45)
pH	7.36	(7.35–7.45)
P_{CO_2}	7.20 kPa	(4.7–6.0)
	54.1 mmHg	(35–45)
P_{O_2}	5.3 kPa	(>10.6)
	40 mmHg	(>80)
Bicarb	30.6 mmol/L	(22–28)
BE	+4.9 mmol/L	(−2 to +2)
S_{O_2}	75.2%	(>96%)
Lactate	1.2 mmol/L	(0.4–1.5)
K	3.7 mmol/L	(3.5–5)
Na	144 mmol/L	(135–145)
Cl	102 mmol/L	(95–105)
iCa^+	1.2 mmol/L	(1–1.25)
Hb	16 g/dL	(13–18)
Glucose	4.9 mmol/L	(3.5–5.5)

Questions

1. a) Describe his gas exchange.
   b) Describe his acid–base status.

2. Which one of the following ABG values is most likely to have changed significantly in the past 24 h: pH, P_{CO_2}, P_{O_2} or HCO_3?

3. Which two of the above ABG values indicate the need for caution when providing O_2 therapy?

CASE 10

History

The patient from Case 9 is treated with nebulised bronchodilators, oral prednisolone and 60% O_2 by face mask. His oxygen saturations improve significantly, but when he is reviewed 1 h later, his condition has deteriorated and he is unable to provide a history.

Examination

He is drowsy and barely rousable. He no longer appears to be in respiratory distress and his respiratory rate has fallen to 14 breaths/min. Chest examination results are unchanged.

Pulse	88 beats/min
Respiratory rate	14 breaths/min
Blood pressure	132/80 mmHg
Sao_2 (room air)	96%

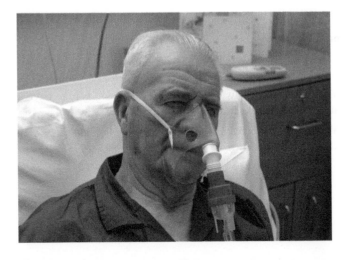

Arterial blood gas		**On 60% O_2**	
23 June 2014			
Unit no.: 00654545			
ID: Hamish R.			
		Normal	
H^+	50.8 nmol/L	(35–45)	
pH	7.29	(7.35–7.45)	
P_{CO_2}	8.7 kPa	(4.7–6.0)	
	65.3 mmHg	(35–45)	
P_{O_2}	11.2 kPa	(>10.6)	
	84.0 mmHg	(>80)	
Bicarb	30.3 mmol/L	(22–28)	
BE	+4.7 mmol/L	(–2 to +2)	
S_{O_2}	96.2%	(>96%)	
Lactate	1.2 mmol/L	(0.4–1.5)	
K	3.6 mmol/L	(3.5–5)	
Na	144 mmol/L	(135–145)	
Cl	102 mmol/L	(95–105)	
iCa^+	1.2 mmol/L	(1–1.25)	
Hb	16 g/dL	(13–18)	
Glucose	5.0 mmol/L	(3.5–5.5)	

Questions

1. a) Describe his gas exchange.
   b) Describe his acid–base status.
2. What has been the cause of his deterioration?

CASE 11

History

A 21-year-old woman presents to the emergency department with a 6-h history of worsening breathlessness and wheeze. She has a history of asthma, with two previous exacerbations requiring hospital admission. She now feels very breathless and is obtaining no relief from her salbutamol inhaler.

Examination

She is tachypnoeic at 30 breaths/min, is using her accessory muscles of respiration and only just managing to speak in full sentences.

Auscultation of her chest reveals widespread polyphonic wheeze.

Pulse	115 beats/min
Blood pressure	120/80 mmHg
SpO_2	96% (room air)
Peak expiratory flow	160 L/s (predicted = 400 L/s)

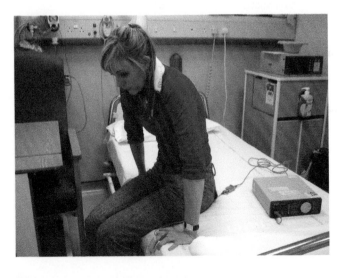

Arterial blood gas 12 Nov. 2013 Unit no.: 12639943 ID: Jessica G.		**On air**
		Normal
H^+	42 nmol/L	(35–45)
pH	7.38	(7.35–7.45)
P_{CO_2}	5.8 kPa	(4.7–6.0)
	43 mmHg	(35–45)
P_{O_2}	10.2 kPa	(>10.6)
	76 mmHg	(>80)
Bicarb	24 mmol/L	(22–28)
BE	−1.3 mmol/L	(−2 to +2)
S_{O_2}	96%	(>96%)
Lactate	1 mmol/L	(0.4–1.5)
K	4.0 mmol/L	(3.5–5)
Na	140 mmol/L	(135–145)
Cl	99 mmol/L	(95–105)
iCa^+	1.12 mmol/L	(1–1.25)
Hb	13.0 g/dL	(11.5–16)
Glucose	5 mmol/L	(3.5–5.5)

Questions

1. a) Describe her gas exchange.
   b) Describe her acid–base status.
2. Which of the above ABG value gives the greatest cause for concern?
3. How would you classify the severity of this asthma attack?

CASE 12

History

A 23-year-old woman presents to the emergency department with a painful ankle, following a simple trip. While being examined by the emergency department doctor she becomes extremely agitated and upset. Despite a normal ankle X-ray and extensive reassurance by the emergency department staff, she refuses to believe that her ankle is not broken and starts crying. While leaving the department, she develops a clutching sensation in her chest, shortness of breath and a tingling sensation in her hands and around her mouth. She reports that she feels unable to take a deep breath.

Examination

The patient appears frightened and extremely distressed. Other than tachypnoea and a mild sinus tachycardia, cardiorespiratory examination is unremarkable. Electrocardiogram, chest X-ray and peak flow measurements are all normal.

Pulse	96 beats/min
Respiratory rate	36 breaths/min
Blood pressure	130/80 mmHg
SpO_2	100%

Arterial blood gas	**On air**	
12 Dec. 2013		
Unit no.: 12534943		
ID: Trinny F.		
		Normal
H^+	29 nmol/L	(35–45)
pH	7.53	(7.35–7.45)
P_{CO_2}	3.14 kPa	(4.7–6.0)
	24 mmHg	(35–45)
P_{O_2}	14.3 kPa	(>10.6)
	108 mmHg	(>80)
Bicarb	24 mmol/L	(22–28)
BE	−1.8 mmol/L	(−2 to +2)
S_{O_2}	99%	(>96%)
Lactate	1 mmol/L	(0.4–1.5)
K	3.5 mmol/L	(3.5–5)
Na	140 mmol/L	(135–145)
Cl	99 mmol/L	(95–105)
iCa^+	0.9 mmol/L	(1–1.25)
Hb	12.0 g/dL	(11.5–16)
Glucose	5 mmol/L	(3.5–5.5)

Questions

1. a) Describe her gas exchange.
   b) Describe her acid–base status.
2. Are there any other abnormalities?
3. What is the likely diagnosis?

CASE 13

History

A 40-year-old man is pulled from a house fire and brought to the emergency department in the early hours of the morning. The paramedics estimate he is likely to have been trapped in a smoke-filled room for up to 20 minutes before rescue.

Examination

The patient is heavily contaminated with soot and smells strongly of smoke. Fortunately, he has not sustained any thermal injuries. He appears to be confused and has just vomited.

Baseline observations are normal, with an oxygen saturation of 99% on 15 L O_2 by mask.

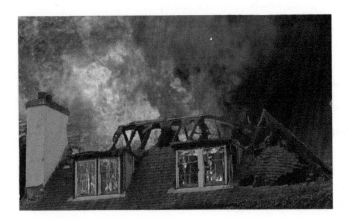

Arterial blood gas
10 Aug. 2014
Unit no.: 77634566
ID: Robert J.

On 15 L O_2 by mask

		Normal
H^+	44 nmol/L	(35–45)
pH	7.36	(7.35–7.45)
PCO_2	4.5 kPa	(4.7–6.0)
	34 mmHg	(35–45)
PO_2	47 kPa	(>10.6)
	353 mmHg	(>80)
Bicarb	18 mmol/L	(22–28)
BE	−5.5 mmol/L	(−2 to +2)
SO_2	100%	(>96%)
Lactate	2 mmol/L	(0.4–1.5)
K	3.6 mmol/L	(3.5–5)
Na	145 mmol/L	(135–145)
Cl	103 mmol/L	(95–105)
iCa^+	1.1 mmol/L	(1–1.25)
Hb	14 g/dL	(13–18)
Glucose	4 mmol/L	(3.5–5.5)

Carbon monoxide assay

CO	40%	(non-smokers < 3%)
		(smokers < 10%)

Questions

1. a) Describe his gas exchange.
   b) Describe his acid–base status.
2. What is the most likely diagnosis?
3. Which of the values provided is *falsely high:* PO_2, SO_2 or Hb?

CASE 14

History

A 68-year-old man is admitted to the emergency department after waking from sleep with severe breathlessness. He was discharged from hospital 4 weeks before after sustaining a large myocardial infarction. Since then he has had no chest pain but has reported gradually worsening breathlessness associated with progressive swelling of the ankles.

Examination

He is in severe respiratory distress and using accessory muscles of respiration. The jugular venous pressure (JVP) is elevated to the earlobe and he has bilateral lower limb oedema to the knees. There are bilateral crackles to the mid zones. His chest X-ray is shown below.

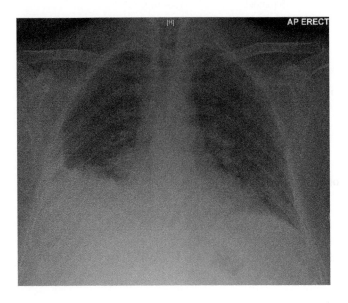

Pulse	128 beats/min
Respiratory rate	40 breaths/min
Blood pressure	144/70 mmHg
Sao_2 (15 L O_2)	91%

Arterial blood gas   **On 15 L O_2 by reservoir mask**
23 Sep. 2014
Unit no.: 00654545
ID: Keegan C.

		Normal
H^+	63 nmol/L	(35–45)
pH	7.21	(7.35–7.45)
Pco_2	6.12 kPa	(4.7–6.0)
	46 mmHg	(35–45)
Po_2	9.3 kPa	(>10.6)
	70 mmHg	(>80)
Bicarb	17.2 mmol/L	(22–28)
BE	–5.9 mmol/L	(–2 to +2)
So_2	93%	(>96%)
Lactate	4.9 mmol/L	(0.4–1.5)
K	3.7 mmol/L	(3.5–5)
Na	141 mmol/L	(135–145)
Cl	100 mmol/L	(95–105)
iCa^+	1.05 mmol/L	(1–1.25)
Hb	16 g/dL	(13–18)
Glucose	8.5 mmol/L	(3.5–5.5)

Questions

1. a) Describe his gas exchange.
   b) Describe his acid–base status.
2. What is the likely diagnosis?
3. What is the cause of the metabolic acid–base disturbance? What factors are driving it?

CASE 15

The patient from Case 14 is treated with a bolus dose of intravenous diuretic and an intravenous infusion of glyceryl trinitrate. After 30 minutes, his Spo_2 has improved but he remains very breathless and appears extremely tired. A repeat blood gas is performed.

Pulse	118 beats/min
Respiratory rate	36 breaths/min
Blood pressure	106/68 mmHg
Spo_2 (15 L O_2)	96%

Arterial blood gas	**On 15 L O_2 by reservoir mask**	
23 Sep. 2014		
Unit no.: 00654545		
ID: Keegan C.		
		Normal
H^+	58 nmol/L	(35–45)
pH	7.24	(7.35–7.45)
P_{CO_2}	6.4 kPa	(4.7–6.0)
	48 mmHg	(35–45)
P_{O_2}	10.7 kPa	(>10.6)
	80 mmHg	(>80)
Bicarb	20.7 mmol/L	(22–28)
BE	–2.9 mmol/L	(–2 to +2)
S_{O_2}	96%	(>96%)
Lactate	3.2 mmol/L	(0.4–1.5)
K	3.5 mmol/L	(3.5–5)
Na	144 mmol/L	(135–145)
Cl	102 mmol/L	(95–105)
iCa^+	1.02 mmol/L	(1–1.25)
Hb	16.5 g/dL	(13–18)
Glucose	9.1 mmol/L	(3.5–5.5)

Questions

1. a) Describe his gas exchange.
   b) Describe his acid–base status.
2. What is the most concerning ABG result?
3. What treatments should be considered now?

CASE 16

History

A 79-year-old woman has just been admitted to the general surgical ward to have a large bowel tumour surgically removed.

The tumour was discovered at colonoscopy after she presented to her doctor with a 6-month history of rectal bleeding.

On admission, she appears to be severely short of breath and extremely tired. Further questioning reveals that her rectal blood loss has been no greater than usual.

Pulse	100 beats/min
Blood pressure	100/80 mmHg
Respiratory rate	24 breaths/min
SaO_2% (on air)	100%

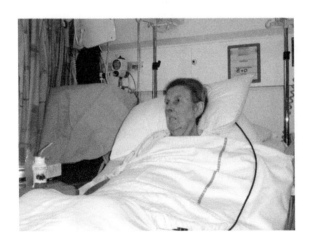

Arterial blood gas		**On air**
06 June 2014		
Unit no.: 943778		
ID: Ethel S.		
		Normal
H^+	32.3 nmol/L	(35–45)
pH	7.49	(7.35–7.45)
P_{CO_2}	3.31 kPa	(4.7–6.0)
	25 mmHg	(35–45)
P_{O_2}	11.9 kPa	(>10.6)
	89 mmHg	(>80)
Bicarb	22 mmol/L	(22–28)
BE	−2 mmol/L	(−2 to +2)
S_{O_2}	99.8%	(>96%)
Lactate	1 mmol/L	(0.4–1.5)
K	3.8 mmol/L	(3.5–5)
Na	138 mmol/L	(135–145)
Cl	96 mmol/L	(95–105)
iCa^+	1.17 mmol/L	(1–1.25)
Hb	6.8 g/dL	(11.5–16)
Glucose	3.9 mmol/L	(3.5–5.5)

Questions

1. a) Describe her gas exchange.
   b) Describe her acid–base state.
2. What is the most likely cause of her breathlessness?
3. What would be the most effective way of improving O_2 delivery to her tissues?

CASE 17

History

A 78-year-old woman is admitted to the emergency department with sudden-onset, generalised, severe, abdominal pain. She describes the pain as being colicky with no particular radiation. She does not complain of any alteration in her bowel habit and has not vomited. Her only medical history is that of atrial fibrillation, for which she takes aspirin and digoxin.

Examination

On examination, the patient is haemodynamically stable with warm, well-perfused peripheries. Despite severe abdominal discomfort, abdominal examination is relatively unremarkable: the abdomen is soft in all four quadrants and is tender only on deep palpation. No hernias or aneurysms are palpable and rectal examination is unremarkable.

An abdominal and erect chest X-ray are taken and found to be normal.

During the course of the examination, her clinical condition deteriorates and she is moved to the resuscitation area.

Arterial blood gas		**On 10 L O$_2$ by mask**
10 Aug. 2014		
Unit no.: 7734211		
ID: Susan U.		
		Normal
H$^+$	52.5 nmol/L	(35–45)
pH	7.28	(7.35–7.45)
P$_{CO_2}$	4.39 kPa	(4.7–6.0)
	33 mmHg	(35–45)
P$_{O_2}$	28.6 kPa	(>10.6)
	215 mmHg	(>80)
Bicarb	16.2 mmol/L	(22–28)
BE	−10.4 mmol/L	(−2 to +2)
S$_{O_2}$	99.8%	(>96%)
Lactate	3.2 mmol/L	(0.4–1.5)
K	4.6 mmol/L	(3.5–5)
Na	135 mmol/L	(135–145)
Cl	96 mmol/L	(95–105)
iCa$^+$	1.16 mmol/L	(1–1.25)
Hb	12 g/dL	(11.5–16)
Glucose	3.8 mmol/L	(3.5–5.5)

Questions

1. a) Describe her gas exchange.
   b) Describe her acid–base status.
2. What is the most likely diagnosis?

CASE 18

History

A 35-year-old woman with type 1 diabetes is brought to the emergency department by ambulance after being found severely unwell in her house. Following a discussion with her partner it emerges she has not been eating for the past few days due to a vomiting illness and, as a precaution, has also been omitting her insulin.

Examination

On examination, she appears drowsy and peripherally shutdown, with very dry mucous membranes. Her breath smells of acetone and her respirations are deep and sighing.

Pulse	130 beats/min
Blood pressure	100/60 mmHg
Respiratory rate	26 breaths/min
BM (blood glucose)	>25 mmol/L

Physical examination of her chest and abdomen is unremarkable.

Arterial blood gas		**On 10 L O$_2$ by mask**
27 Feb. 2014		
Unit no.: 77735566		
ID: Isla T.		
		Normal
H$^+$	88.9 nmol/L	(35–45)
pH	7.05	(7.35–7.45)
P$_{CO_2}$	1.5 kPa	(4.7–6.0)
	11 mmHg	(35–45)
P$_{O_2}$	28.4 kPa	(>10.6)
	187 mmHg	(>80)
Bicarb	6.0 mmol/L	(22–28)
BE	−25.2 mmol/L	(−2 to +2)
S$_{O_2}$	99.8%	(>96%)
Lactate	1 mmol/L	(0.4–1.5)
K	4.6 mmol/L	(3.5–5)
Na	141 mmol/L	(135–145)
Cl	96 mmol/L	(95–105)
iCa$^+$	1.25 mmol/L	(1–1.25)
Hb	12 g/dL	(11.5–16)
Glucose	35 mmol/L	(3.5–5.5)

Questions

1. a) Describe her gas exchange.
   b) Describe her acid–base status.
2. Calculate the anion gap.
3. What is the most likely diagnosis?

CASE 19

History

A 37-year-old well-known local vagrant is brought into the department unconscious. He was found near a bottle of vodka and a half-empty bottle of what appears to be methanol. It is unclear if he has drunk any of the contents.

Examination

The patient is unkempt, with a significantly reduced conscious level (Glasgow Coma Scale score = 9). There are no apparent focal neurological abnormalities.

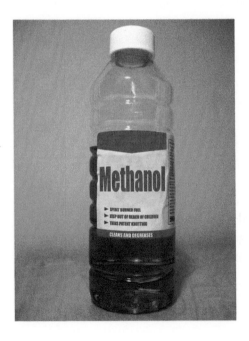

Arterial blood gas		**On air**
10 July 2014		
Unit no.: 35477899		
ID: Gary S.		
		Normal
H$^+$	63.3 nmol/L	(35–45)
pH	7.20	(7.35–7.45)
P_{CO_2}	3.3 kPa	(4.7–6.0)
	25 mmHg	(35–45)
P_{O_2}	12.8 kPa	(>10.6)
	96 mmHg	(>80)
Bicarb	9.5 mmol/L	(22–28)
BE	−16.2 mmol/L	(−2 to +2)
S_{O_2}	97.8%	(>96%)
Lactate	1.3 mmol/L	(0.4–1.5)
K	4.5 mmol/L	(3.5–5)
Na	136 mmol/L	(135–145)
Cl	99 mmol/L	(95–105)
iCa$^+$	1.1 mmol/L	(1–1.25)
Hb	13.5 g/dL	(13–18)
Glucose	3.8 mmol/L	(3.5–5.5)

Questions

1. a) Describe his gas exchange.
    b) Describe his acid–base status.
2. What is the anion gap?
3. Is the acid–base status consistent with methanol ingestion?

CASE 20

History

A 52-year-old man is being investigated on the urology ward for recurrent renal stones (arrow). He also complains of mild fatigue and lethargy. There is no history of gastrointestinal disturbance and he is not on any regular medications.

Examination

The patient is well and clinical examination reveals no abnormalities.

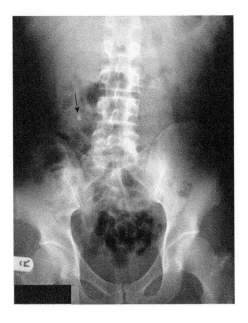

As part of the investigations, an ABG is obtained.

Arterial blood gas		**On air**
23 Apr. 2014		
Unit no.: 27634943		
ID: Roger P.		
		Normal
H^+	43 nmol/L	(35–45)
pH	7.37	(7.35–7.45)
P_{CO_2}	4.2 kPa	(4.7–6.0)
	31.5 mmHg	(35–45)
P_{O_2}	13.2 kPa	(>10.6)
	99.0 mmHg	(>80)
Bicarb	18 mmol/L	(22–28)
BE	–7 mmol/L	(–2 to +2)
S_{O_2}	99%	(>96%)
Lactate	1 mmol/L	(0.4–1.5)
K	3.0 mmol/L	(3.5–5)
Na	137 mmol/L	(135–145)
Cl	109 mmol/L	(95–105)
iCa^+	1.0 mmol/L	(1–1.25)
Hb	13.0 g/dL	(13–18)
Glucose	4 mmol/L	(3.5–5.5)

Questions

1. a) Describe his gas exchange.
   b) Describe his acid–base status.
2. Calculate the anion gap.
3. What is the most likely diagnosis?

CASE 21

History

An 18-year-old is admitted to the toxicology unit having taken a large overdose of an unknown substance 5 h earlier. She complains of nausea and a high-pitched noise in her ears.

Examination

On examination, she is mildly confused. Her respirations are increased in both rate and depth. Examination is otherwise unremarkable.

Pulse	100 beats/min
Respiratory rate	26 breaths/min
Blood pressure	132/100 mmHg
Temperature	37.6°C
O_2%	99%

Arterial blood gas		**On air**
10 Sep. 2014		
Unit no.: 27634943		
ID: Libby F.		
		Normal
H^+	38.8 nmol/L	(35–45)
pH	7.41	(7.35–7.45)
P_{CO_2}	3.01 kPa	(4.7–6.0)
	22.6 mmHg	(35–45)
P_{O_2}	14.1 kPa	(>10.6)
	97.5 mmHg	(>80)
Bicarb	17.6 mmol/L	(22–28)
BE	−8.3 mmol/L	(−2 to +2)
S_{O_2}	99%	(>96%)
Lactate	1.4 mmol/L	(0.4–1.5)
K	3.6 mmol/L	(3.5–5)
Na	140 mmol/L	(135–145)
Cl	99 mmol/L	(95–105)
iCa^+	1.2 mmol/L	(1–1.25)
Hb	13.0 g/dL	(11.5–16)
Glucose	5 mmol/L	(3.5–5.5)

Questions

1. a) Describe her gas exchange.
   b) Describe her acid–base status.
2. Calculate the anion gap.
3. What substance is she most likely to have taken?

CASE 22

History

A 64-year-old woman is referred to critical care after becoming unwell 48 h after an invasive urology procedure.

Examination

She appears flushed and sweaty, with a pyrexia of 39.8°C. She has a sinus tachycardia of 122 beats/min and a blood pressure of 100/65 mmHg. C-reactive protein is elevated at 267 mg/dL. Her observation chart and ABG results are shown below.

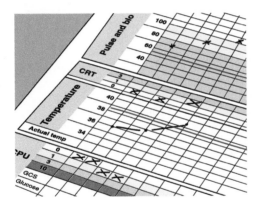

Arterial blood gas		**On 10 L O$_2$**
11 July 2014		
Unit no.: 37564349		
ID: Sonia K.		
		Normal
H$^+$	13.5 nmol/L	(35–45)
pH	7.36	(7.35–7.45)
PCO_2	4.2 kPa	(4.7–6.0)
	31.5 mmHg	(35–45)
PO_2	27.1 kPa	(>10.6)
	203 mmHg	(>80)
Bicarb	17.3 mmol/L	(22–28)
BE	−6.9 mmol/L	(−2 to +2)
SO_2	100%	(>96%)
Lactate	5.1 mmol/L	(0.4–1.5)
K	4.1 mmol/L	(3.5–5)
Na	140 mmol/L	(135–145)
Cl	101 mmol/L	(95–105)
iCa$^+$	1.1 mmol/L	(1–1.25)
Hb	15.0 g/dL	(11.5–16)
Glucose	6.8 mmol/L	(3.5–5.5)

Questions

1. a) Describe her gas exchange.
   b) Describe her acid–base status.
2. What is the cause of the acid–base abnormality?
3. Which ABG value carries the greatest significance for prognosis and treatment in this context?

CASE 23

History

A 24-year-old man is brought to hospital by his family after becoming unwell at home. They report that he has no history of significant medical illness but has recently been undergoing tests for progressive fatigue and weight loss. Over the last few days, he has become increasingly weak and lethargic and has also complained of muscle cramps. They became alarmed today when he appeared drowsy and disoriented.

Examination

The patient appears listless and confused. He has cool peripheries and poor capillary refill. He is afebrile and there is no rash, lymphadenopathy or meningism. Abdominal examination is unremarkable and there are no focal chest or neurological signs.

Pulse	120 beats/min
Respiratory rate	25 breaths/min
Blood pressure	75/55 mmHg
Temperature	36.5°C
BM (blood glucose)	2.9 mmol/L

Arterial blood gas	**On air**	
10 Aug. 2014		
Unit no.: 456986793		
ID: Rufus W.		
		Normal
H$^+$	48 nmol/L	(35–45)
pH	7.32	(7.35–7.45)
PCO_2	3.3 kPa	(4.7–6.0)
	24.8 mmHg	(35–45)
PO_2	13 kPa	(>10.6)
	97 mmHg	(>80)
Bicarb	13.4 mmol/L	(22–28)
BE	−13.9 mmol/L	(−2 to +2)
SO_2	99%	(>96%)
Lactate	3 mmol/L	(0.4–1.5)
K	5.6 mmol/L	(3.5–5)
Na	125 mmol/L	(135–145)
Cl	101 mmol/L	(95–105)
iCa$^+$	1.2 mmol/L	(1–1.25)
Hb	13.0 g/dL	(13–18)
Glucose	2.5 mmol/L	(3.5–5.5)

Questions

1. a) Describe his gas exchange.
   b) Describe his acid–base state.
2. Are there any other abnormalities on the ABG?
3. What specific treatment does this patient require?

CASE 24

History

An 87-year-old man has been found collapsed in the ward toilet. Cardiopulmonary resuscitation was commenced promptly, as no pulse or respiratory effort was detected, and has now been in progress for 12 minutes. He has a medical history of ischaemic heart disease, dementia and chronic renal failure.

Examination

The patient has a Glasgow Coma Scale score of 3 and appears pale and mottled. The cardiac monitor reveals an agonal rhythm as shown below. No pulses are palpable and there is no respiratory effort. He is currently being ventilated by a bag and mask on 15 L/min of O_2.

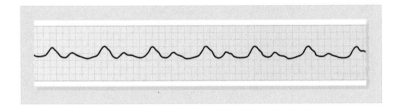

Arterial blood gas		**On 15 L O_2 by bag and mask**
10 Feb. 2014		
Unit no.: 42333993		
ID: David K.		
		Normal
H'	160 nmol/L	(35–45)
pH	6.8	(7.35–7.45)
P_{CO_2}	4.8 kPa	(4.7–6.0)
	36 mmHg	(35–45)
P_{O_2}	32 kPa	(>10.6)
	240 mmHg	(>80)
Bicarb	3.8 mmol/L	(22–28)
BE	–20 mmol/L	(–2 to +2)
S_{O_2}	100%	(>96%)
Lactate	9 mmol/L	(0.4–1.5)
K	4.5 mmol/L	(3.5–5)
Na	136 mmol/L	(135–145)
Cl	96 mmol/L	(95–105)
Ca^+	1.1 mmol/L	(1–1.25)
Hb	14.0 g/dL	(13–18)
Glucose	4 mmol/L	(3.5–5.5)

Questions

1. a) Describe his gas exchange.
   b) Describe his acid–base status.
2. What is his prognosis?

CASE 25

History

A 59-year-old man with a history of alcohol excess presents to the emergency department with a 3-day history of severe upper abdominal pain. He now also feels very breathless. He admits to drinking up to 100 units of alcohol per week for the past few weeks.

Examination

The patient is in evident distress and appears very unwell. He is tachycardic (120 beats/min) and hypotensive (75/60 mmHg). There is marked epigastric tenderness.

A venous blood test taken on admission reveals a grossly elevated amylase (1890 U/mL) and C-reactive protein (274 mg/L). A chest X-ray on admission is shown below.

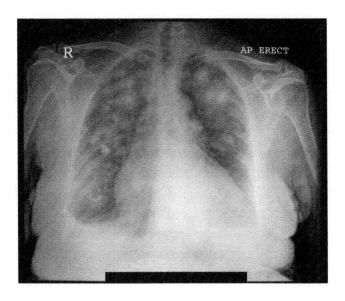

Arterial blood gas 10 Aug. 2014 Unit no.: 45679393 ID: Daniel C.	**On 15 L O_2 by mask with reservoir bag**	
		Normal
H^+	49 nmol/l	(35–45)
pH	7.33	(7.35–7.45)
P_{CO_2}	3.51 kPa	(4.7–6.0)
	24.3 mmHg	(35–45)
P_{O_2}	10.8 kPa	(>10.6)
	81 mmHg	(>80)
Bicarb	12.9 mmol/L	(22–28)
BE	−11.8 mmol/L	(−2 to +2)
S_{O_2}	99%	(>96%)
Lactate	3.1 mmol/L	(0.4–1.5)
K	3.6 mmol/L	(3.5–5)
Na	141 mmol/L	(135–145)
Cl	96 mmol/L	(95–105)
iCa^+	0.89 mmol/L	(1–1.25)
Hb	12.0 g/dL	(13–18)
Glucose	16 mmol/L	(3.5–5.5)

Questions

1. a) Describe his gas exchange.
   b) Describe his acid–base status.
2. What is his approximate F_{IO_2}?
3. What is the most likely diagnosis?

CASE 26

History

A 35-year-old woman on a gynaecology ward develops a severe vomiting illness 1 day after elective sterilisation. She continues to vomit profusely for another 3 days. Examination of her fluid balance chart reveals that she is failing to keep up with her fluid losses but has not been prescribed intravenous fluids.

Examination

The patient appears dehydrated, with reduced skin turgor and dry mucous membranes.

Abdominal examination is unremarkable.

Pulse	100 beats/min
Respiratory rate	10 breaths/min
Blood pressure	160/100 mmHg
Temperature	36.6°C
O_2%	96%

Arterial blood gas		**On air**	
23 Aug. 2014			
Unit no.: 27634943			
ID: Jenny A.			
		Normal	
H^+	36 nmol/L	(35–45)	
pH	7.44	(7.35–7.45)	
P_{CO_2}	6.4 kPa	(4.7–6.0)	
	48 mmHg	(35–45)	
P_{O_2}	11.1 kPa	(>10.6)	
	83 mmHg	(>80)	
Bicarb	32 mmol/L	(22–28)	
BE	+4 mmol/L	(–2 to +2)	
S_{O_2}	96%	(>96%)	
Lactate	1 mmol/L	(0.4–1.5)	
K	3.0 mmol/L	(3.5–5)	
Na	133 mmol/L	(135–145)	
Cl	91 mmol/L	(95–105)	
iCa^+	1.0 mmol/L	(1–1.25)	
Hb	11.0 g/dL	(11.5–16)	
Glucose	5 mmol/L	(3.5–5.5)	

Questions

1. a) Describe her gas exchange.
   b) Describe her acid–base status.
2. What electrolyte abnormalities are present?
3. What treatment will correct the acid–base abnormality?

CASE 27

History

An 8-week-old child is brought to the emergency department, with weight loss and projectile vomiting. The parents report that he had an uncomplicated delivery with no postpartum complications. He initially fed well, appeared to be thriving and gave no cause for concern but has deteriorated markedly over the past 2 weeks, vomiting all of his meals and now losing weight.

Examination

The child is agitated, crying and malnourished. His mucous membranes are dry, and on examination of his abdomen, a small mass is found in the epigastrium.

Capillary blood gas	**On air**	
05 Oct. 2013		
Unit no.: 28734943		
ID: Richard B.		
		Normal
H$^+$	20 nmol/L	(35–45)
pH	7.54	(7.35–7.45)
P_{CO_2}	6.1 kPa	(4.7–6.0)
	45.8 mmHg	(35–45)
P_{O_2}	11.2 kPa	(>10.6)
	80 mmHg	(>80)
Bicarb	37.5 mmol/L	(22–28)
BE	+14 mmol/L	(–2 to +2)
S_{O_2}	99%	(>96%)
Lactate	1 mmol/L	(0.4–1.5)
K	2.5 mmol/L	(3.5–5)
Na	135 mmol/L	(135–145)
Cl	86 mmol/L	(95–105)
iCa$^+$	1 mmol/L	(1–1.25)
Hb	18.0 g/dL	(13–18)
Glucose	5.1 mmol/L	(3.5–5.5)

Questions

1. a) Describe his gas exchange.
   b) Describe his acid–base status.

2. Considering the pH and HCO$_3$, is the Pa_{CO_2} higher or lower than you would expect?

3. What is the underlying diagnosis?

CASE 28

History

A 69-year-old woman with advanced chronic obstructive pulmonary disease and severe right heart failure (cor pulmonale) is receiving inpatient treatment with intravenous diuretics for worsening peripheral oedema, resistant to high-dose oral therapy. There has been no recent change in breathlessness or sputum production.

Examination

She has evidence of chest hyperinflation and globally diminished breath sounds. Her JVP is markedly elevated and there is extensive peripheral oedema with ascites. She does not appear in respiratory distress.

Pulse	90 beats/min
Respiratory rate	16 breaths/min
Blood pressure	136/80 mmHg
Sao_2	90% (on room air)
Temperature	36.3°C

Arterial blood gas		**On room air**
11 July 2014		
Unit no.: 779624389		
ID: Margaret M.		
		Normal
H$^+$	32.2 nmol/L	(35–45)
pH	7.49	(7.35–7.45)
PCO_2	6.9 kPa	(4.7–6.0)
	51.8 mmHg	(35–45)
PO_2	7.6 kPa	(>10.6)
	57 mmHg	(>80)
Bicarb	38 mmol/L	(22–28)
BE	+6.8 mmol/L	(–2 to +2)
SO_2	89%	(>96%)
Lactate	1.3 mmol/L	(0.4–1.5)
K	3.0 mmol/L	(3.5–5)
Na	131 mmol/L	(135–145)
Cl	88 mmol/L	(95–105)
iCa$^+$	1.0 mmol/L	(1–1.25)
Hb	17.7 g/dL	(11.5–16)
Glucose	5.8 mmol/L	(3.5–5.5)

Questions

1. a) Describe her gas exchange.
   b) Describe her acid–base status.
2. What treatment might help to improve the acid–base abnormality?

CASE 29

History

A 36-year-old pregnant woman on the maternity ward complains of feeling short of breath. She has no other symptoms and no relevant medical history.

Examination

On examination, the patient is heavily pregnant but appears otherwise well. Examination of her chest reveals no abnormalities.

Pulse	110 beats/min
Respiratory rate	20 breaths/min
Blood pressure	112/100 mmHg
Temperature	36.6°C
O_2%	99%

An ABG is performed.

Arterial blood gas		**On air**	
18 Mar. 2014			
Unit no.: 27634943			
ID: Julie D.			
		Normal	
H'	35 nmol/L	(35–45)	
pH	7.45	(7.35–7.45)	
P_{CO_2}	4.9 kPa	(4.7–6.0)	
	37 mmHg	(35–45)	
P_{O_2}	4.7 kPa	(>10.6)	
	35 mmHg	(>80)	
Bicarb	24.0 mmol/L	(22–28)	
BE	2 mmol/L	(−2 to +2)	
S_{O_2}	74%	(>96%)	
Lactate	1 mmol/L	(0.4–1.5)	
K	3.6 mmol/L	(3.5–5)	
Na	138 mmol/L	(135–145)	
Cl	104 mmol/L	(95–105)	
iCa^+	1.14 mmol/L	(1–1.25)	
Hb	13.0 g/dL	(11.5–16)	
Glucose	5 mmol/L	(3.5–5.5)	

Questions

1. a) Describe her gas exchange.
   b) Describe her acid–base status.
2. What is the most likely explanation for the low P_{O_2}?

CASE 30

History

A 55-year-old woman on the orthopaedic ward complains of sudden-onset breathlessness and pain on the left-hand side of her chest. She underwent elective knee replacement surgery 4 days before and has been immobile in bed since the operation. She is otherwise well with no relevant medical history.

Examination

The patient appears well but slightly short of breath. Other than mild tachycardia and tachypnoea, examination of the cardiovascular and respiratory systems yields no positive findings, and there is no clinical evidence of deep-vein thrombosis.

A chest X-ray reveals no abnormalities and an electrocardiogram shows only sinus tachycardia.

Pulse	98 beats/min
Respiratory rate	20 breaths/min
Blood pressure	160/100 mmHg
Temperature	36.6°C
O_2%	99%

Arterial blood gas	**On air**	
10 May 2014		
Unit no.: 27634943		
ID: Jill A.		
		Normal
H^+	36 nmol/L	(35–45)
pH	7.43	(7.35–7.45)
P_{CO_2}	4.9 kPa	(4.7–6.0)
	37 mmHg	(35–45)
P_{O_2}	12.1 kPa	(>10.6)
	91 mmHg	(>80)
Bicarb	25.8 mmol/L	(22–28)
BE	−1.8 mmol/L	(−2 to +2)
S_{O_2}	99%	(>96%)
Lactate	1 mmol/L	(0.4–1.5)
K	3.8 mmol/L	(3.5–5)
Na	136 mmol/L	(135–145)
Cl	99 mmol/L	(95–105)
iCa^+	1.2 mmol/L	(1–1.25)
Hb	10.0 g/dL	(11.5–16)
Glucose	5 mmol/L	(3.5–5.5)

Questions

1. a) Describe her gas exchange.
   b) Describe her acid–base status.
2. What is the A – a gradient?
3. Does she require any further investigation?

ANSWERS

1. a) Type 1 respiratory impairment (moderate)
   b) Uncompensated respiratory alkalosis
2. Yes
3. Yes

This patient has moderate type 1 respiratory impairment. Although hyperventilation is an appropriate response to the hypoxaemia and sensation of dyspnoea, it has resulted in a mild alkalaemia (remember that metabolic compensation does not occur in response to *acute* respiratory acid–base disturbance).

The correct management for his condition is supplemental oxygen to correct the hypoxaemia and appropriate antibiotics to treat the infection.

In a patient such as this, with moderate hypoxaemia and no ventilatory impairment, monitoring by pulse oximetry is more appropriate than repeated ABG sampling. Indications for further ABG analysis would include signs of exhaustion or hypercapnia (p. 23) or a further significant decline in Sao_2.

CASE 2

1. a) Chronic type 2 respiratory impairment
   b) Compensated respiratory acidosis
2. Chronic type 2 respiratory impairment due to morbid obesity

At first glance, it may be difficult to determine whether this ABG represents respiratory acidosis with metabolic compensation or metabolic alkalosis with respiratory compensation, as both give a high HCO_3 and a high $Pa\text{CO}_2$ level. The best clue is the pH (or H^+) which, although just within the normal range, is on the brink of acidaemia. This would represent overcompensation for an alkalosis and, therefore, suggests an acidosis as the *primary* abnormality (overcompensation does not occur). The mildly impaired oxygenation is consistent with the degree of hypoventilation.

The most likely cause of chronic type 2 respiratory impairment in this case is severe obesity. Approximately 20% of individuals with a body mass index greater than 40 have chronic hypercapnia from restricted ventilation (pickwickian syndrome).

CASE 3

1. a) Mild type 1 respiratory impairment (with marked hyperventilation)
   b) Uncompensated respiratory alkalosis
2. Pulmonary embolism

This patient is a young, fit, non-smoker with no history of lung problems but, despite hyperventilating (low Pa_{CO_2}), has a Pa_{O_2} below the normal range, indicating impaired oxygenation. Given the recent long-haul flight and absence of clinical and X-ray abnormalities, the most likely cause of her breathlessness and impaired oxygenation is pulmonary embolism, and she must be investigated accordingly.

This is one of the clinical situations where calculation of the A–a gradient can be helpful (more so when the Pa_{O_2} is just within the normal range). As shown below, it is significantly elevated, indicating the presence of $\dot{V}/\dot{Q}$ mismatch.

A – a gradient = $PA_{O_2} - Pa_{O_2}$
$Pa_{O_2} = (0.21 \times 93.8) - (3.9 \times 1.2)$
$\quad = 19.7 - 4.7$
$\quad = 15$ kPa
A – a gradient = $15 - 10.3$
$\quad\quad\quad = 4.7$ (norm <2.6 kPa)

OR

$Pa_{O_2} = (0.21 \times 713) - (29.3 \times 1.2)$
$\quad = 150 - 35$
$\quad = 115$
A – a gradient = $115 - 77$
$\quad\quad\quad = 38$ mmHg (norm <20 mmHg)

CASE 4

1. a) Acute type 2 respiratory failure
   b) Uncompensated respiratory acidosis
2. Opioid toxicity
3. Opioid antagonist

Opioids have a depressant effect on respiration and may lead to acute ventilatory failure (type 2 respiratory failure). This elderly man has received a large amount of morphine in a short period and exhibits pinpoint pupils, making opioid toxicity by far the most likely cause of his severe ventilatory failure. Because metabolic compensation takes several days to occur, the acute respiratory acidosis has produced a severe acidaemia.

His Pa_{O_2}, although within the normal range, is lower than expected for a patient breathing 28% O_2, and more or less consistent with this degree of hypoventilation.

In addition to basic life-support measures, he should be administered an opioid antagonist (e.g. naloxone) to reverse the respiratory depression, and then closely monitored to ensure sustained improvement.

CASE 5

1. a) Type 1 respiratory impairment (moderate)
   b) Normal acid–base balance
2. Yes

The above ABG is helpful in guiding the correct treatment for this patient with acute exacerbation of chronic obstructive pulmonary disease (COPD). Patients with this condition are often prescribed inadequate oxygen for fear of suppressing hypoxic drive (and thereby depressing ventilation), but this is an issue only in patients with *chronic type 2* respiratory failure (indicated by $\uparrow Pa\text{CO}_2$ and $\uparrow \text{HCO}_3$). This patient has *type 1* respiratory impairment and will not rely on hypoxic drive.

Although this patient is likely to have a chronically low $Pa\text{O}_2$, the acute deterioration in both his symptoms and exercise tolerance suggests a further recent decline from his normal baseline. Importantly, even a small drop in $Pa\text{O}_2$ around this level [steep part of the O_2–haemoglobin (Hb) curve] may cause a marked reduction in $Sa\text{O}_2$, compromising O_2 delivery to tissues. Thus, O_2 is required both to alleviate symptoms and to prevent the development of tissue hypoxia, and *should not* be withheld for fear of precipitating hypoventilation.

CASE 6

1. a) Acute type 2 respiratory impairment
   b) Uncompensated respiratory acidosis
2. No!

This patient with an acute exacerbation of COPD has been struggling to overcome severe obstruction to airflow over a period of hours to days and is now exhausted from the increased work of breathing. As a result, his alveolar ventilation is declining, leading to acute type 2 respiratory failure. This may complicate type 1 respiratory failure from any cause, not just from COPD. The rising $Pa\text{CO}_2$ is, therefore, *not* due to diminished hypoxic drive and removing his oxygen will *not* correct it. Indeed, his $Fi\text{O}_2$ should probably be increased (in addition to other treatment) as he remains significantly hypoxaemic.

Remember that, with acute respiratory acidosis, there is no time for metabolic compensation to develop and a dangerous acidaemia develops rapidly. Adequate ventilation must be restored, as a matter of urgency, to correct the $Pa\text{CO}_2$. Possible measures, in this case, include a respiratory stimulant (e.g. doxapram) or, preferably, non-invasive ventilation. If these fail, intubation and mechanical ventilation may be required, if considered appropriate.

CASE 7

1. a) Type 1 respiratory impairment
   b) Normal
2. Long-term home oxygen therapy

Long-term supplementary oxygen therapy for a minimum of 15 h/day has been shown to improve survival in COPD patients with severe hypoxaemia. It should be offered to patients who, despite being clinically stable and on optimal medical therapy, have a Pao_2 less than 7.3 kPa [or <8 kPa if accompanied by secondary polycythaemia, pulmonary hypertension or evidence of right heart failure (e.g. peripheral oedema)]. Ideally, the Pao_2 should be confirmed on two separate ABGs taken at least 3 weeks apart. Because of the significant risk of fire hazard, home oxygen therapy is usually not offered to patients who continue to smoke.

CASE 8

1. a) Type 1 respiratory impairment
   b) Mild respiratory alkalosis balanced by mild metabolic acidosis (likely two primary processes)
2. Aspiration pneumonia
3. Severe

This patient has mild to moderate hypoxaemia despite receiving a high Fio_2, and therefore, has severe impairment of oxygenation. The slightly low $Paco_2$ indicates that ventilation is adequate, so this is type 1 respiratory impairment. The probable explanation for the mild metabolic acidosis is lactic acidosis resulting from tissue hypoxia.

The history, examination findings and chest X-ray all suggest a diagnosis of aspiration pneumonia.

This patient is severely unwell and any further decline in her Pao_2 could be catastrophic (on the steep part of the O_2–Hb saturation curve). Her O_2 therapy should be adjusted as necessary to maintain her Sao_2 above 92% and she should be managed on a high-dependency unit with close monitoring for signs of deterioration.

CASE 9

1. a) Chronic type 2 respiratory impairment
   b) Compensated respiratory acidosis
2. Po_2
3. Pco_2 and HCO_3

Acute exacerbation of COPD is a common medical emergency and this case illustrates key principles:

1. The ↑$Paco_2$ shows the patient has type 2 respiratory impairment (ventilatory impairment).
2. The ↑HCO_3 tells us it is *chronic* type 2 impairment (because metabolic compensation takes time to develop).
3. Even in chronic type 2 impairment, a further *acute* rise in $Paco_2$ would lead to an acidaemia. The pH here is normal, so the $Paco_2$ has not changed appreciably in the last few days (i.e. there is no acute-on-chronic rise).
4. His Pao_2 *is* likely to have dropped, leading to the increased breathlessness and marked decline in exercise capacity: below a Pao_2 of 8 kPa (60 mmHg), even small falls may cause a major decline in Sao_2 (steep part of the curve).
5. As this patient has chronic hypercapnia, he may rely on hypoxic drive as a stimulus to ventilation.
6. The goal is to ensure adequate oxygenation (we must not ignore his hypoxaemia) without depressing ventilatory drive.

CASE 10

1. a) Acute-on-chronic type 2 respiratory impairment
   b) Partially compensated respiratory acidosis
2. Excessive supplemental O_2

Care must be taken when prescribing supplemental O_2 to patients with chronic type 2 respiratory failure. The aim is to reverse any recent worsening of hypoxaemia and allow adequate tissue oxygenation, without depressing ventilatory drive through an excessive rise in Pao_2.

Most authorities recommend controlled O_2 therapy using a fixed-concentration mask at an initial concentration of 24–28%. The response to therapy must be closely monitored, with frequent clinical assessment and repeated ABG measurement. Note that pulse oximetry is *not* an adequate substitute for ABG in these circumstances, as knowledge of the Sao_2 alone does not permit assessment of ventilatory adequacy.

The latter point is well illustrated in this case as the patient now has life-threatening acute-on-chronic respiratory failure despite a normal Sao_2. The rising $Paco_2$ must be rapidly checked and reversed through improving ventilation. Potential strategies include reducing inspired O_2 concentration, respiratory stimulants or assisted ventilation.

CASE 11

1. a) Mild type 1 respiratory impairment
   b) Normal
2. The $Pa\text{CO}_2$ (high end of normal range)
3. Life-threatening attack

This patient has several features of a severe asthma attack but it is the high–normal $Pa\text{CO}_2$ that is the most worrying aspect of her presentation and makes it a life-threatening attack. Patients with acute exacerbations of asthma should have a low $Pa\text{CO}_2$ due to the increased respiratory rate and effort ($\uparrow$alveolar ventilation). A level >5 kPa (37.5 mmHg) suggests that the patient is struggling to overcome the obstruction to airflow and, perhaps, beginning to tire from the effort of breathing. Consequently, her $Pa\text{CO}_2$ signals a life-threatening attack.

The intensive care unit should be informed immediately of any patient with acute severe asthma and life-threatening features. Patients must receive intensive treatment and monitoring, including repeated ABG measurements to assess response and identify the need for intubation.

CASE 12

1. a) Hyperventilation (primary)
   b) Uncompensated respiratory alkalosis
2. Low ionised calcium
3. Psychogenic hyperventilation

This is a classic clinical picture of psychogenic hyperventilation. The ABG is entirely in keeping with this diagnosis as it reveals evidence of hyperventilation (low Pa_{CO_2}) with normal oxygenation (normal Pa_{O_2}) and a normal A – a gradient.

Note that the HCO_3 (and base excess) is normal, as there has been insufficient time for metabolic compensation to occur. Consequently, the reduction in Pa_{CO_2} has caused a marked alkalaemia.

Another point to note is that the concentration of ionised calcium in the blood is affected by the pH of the specimen, because H^+ ions compete with calcium for binding sites on albumin and other proteins. Therefore, as the number of H^+ drops (alkalaemia), more calcium is bound to albumin, causing serum ionised calcium levels to fall. This is the most likely cause of the numbness and tingling.

Care must be taken in ruling out other cardiovascular and respiratory pathologies before ascribing symptoms of chest pain and shortness of breath to psychogenic hyperventilation.

CASE 13

1. a) Normal – but severe hypoxaemia
   b) Compensated metabolic acidosis
2. Carbon monoxide (CO) poisoning
3. So_2

CO poisoning commonly presents with nausea, vomiting, headache and confusion. CO saturations correlate poorly with symptoms but levels above 50% may cause cardiac arrest and seizures.

WHY IS THE PATIENT HYPOXAEMIC?

CO binds to Hb with *200 times* the affinity of O_2 and, therefore, is carried on the Hb molecule (as carboxyhaemoglobin) in preference to O_2. As a consequence, the percentage of Hb saturated with O_2 – the Sao_2 – is markedly reduced in CO poisoning, even when the Pao_2 is very high. Because the overall O_2 content of blood is determined by the Sao_2 and Hb concentration, O_2 delivery to tissues is inadequate (tissue hypoxia), leading to lactic acidosis.

WHY DOES Sao_2 APPEAR TO BE NORMAL?

Most pulse oximeters are unable to distinguish carboxyhaemoglobin from oxyhaemoglobin and, therefore, fail to reflect the true Sao_2 in CO poisoning. In ABG analysis, the So_2 is not normally measured but simply *calculated* from the measured Po_2. The latter parameter is based only on free, unbound O_2 molecules, and so it is unaffected by the presence of CO.

CASE 14

1. a) Type 2 respiratory impairment. Oxygenation severely impaired but adequate on high FiO_2
   b) Mixed respiratory and metabolic acidosis, resulting in severe acidaemia
2. Acute decompensated heart failure with pulmonary oedema
3. Lactic acidosis. Hypoxaemia. Impaired tissue perfusion. Increased respiratory muscle work

This patient has acute pulmonary oedema due to left ventricular failure. Pulmonary oedema is more commonly associated with type 1 respiratory impairment (due to $\dot{V}/\dot{Q}$ mismatch) rather than type 2 respiratory impairment but it is important to remember that exhaustion may lead to ventilatory failure in severe type 1 respiratory impairment from any cause. A PO_2 of 9.3 kPa with an FiO_2 of 0.6–0.8 indicates severely impaired oxygenation and suggests that the patient may have been profoundly hypoxaemic before the administration of O_2 by paramedics. This is likely to be the main driver of his lactic acidosis, although increased O_2 demand from respiratory muscle use and impaired tissue perfusion from impaired cardiac output may also be contributing. This patient is currently on a knife-edge. The elevated $PaCO_2$ suggests he has exhausted his respiratory reserve and the mixed acidosis precludes physiological compensation and is already producing severe acidaemia.

CASE 15

1. a) Worsening type 2 respiratory impairment. Oxygenation severely impaired but adequate on high F_{IO_2}
   b) Severe acidaemia due to mixed metabolic and respiratory acidosis Improving metabolic acidosis but deteriorating respiratory acidosis
2. Rising Pa_{CO_2}
3. Ventilatory support (e.g. intubation and mechanical ventilation)

The patient is now less acidaemic due to the resolving lactic acidosis. This is likely to reflect a sustained improvement in oxygenation (and subsequent O_2 delivery to tissues) following the administration of high-flow O_2 as well as an additional increase in oxygenation from the treatment of pulmonary oedema (reduced $\dot{V}/\dot{Q}$ mismatch). Unfortunately, the overall trend in acid–base status masks a concerning increase in respiratory acidosis. The worsening ventilatory failure is almost certainly due to exhaustion from the very high work of breathing. Continued aggressive treatment of the pulmonary oedema may help to relieve the work of breathing, but this patient is likely to require ventilatory support (e.g. tracheal intubation), at least in the short term.

CASE 16

1. a) Hyperventilation – no impairment of oxygenation but hypoxaemia secondary to anaemia (p. 18)
    b) Uncompensated respiratory alkalosis
2. Anaemia (Hb = 6.8 g/dL)
3. Restore Hb concentration (e.g. blood transfusion, iron replacement)

This patient appears to have severe anaemia, most likely due to iron deficiency from chronic rectal bleeding. This should be confirmed with a formal laboratory sample (full blood count).

There is no impairment of ventilation or O_2 transfer and, therefore, Pao_2 and Sao_2 are normal. However, the vast majority of O_2 in blood is carried by Hb, so the overall O_2 *content* of her blood is low.

Hyperventilation is a normal response to the sensation of breathlessness and increases the Pao_2 slightly. However, in the aforementioned context, this has very little impact on blood O_2 content, as the available Hb molecules are already fully saturated.

For the same reason, supplemental O_2 would also fail to improve O_2 content significantly. Indeed, the only effective strategy is to increase Hb concentration. This could be achieved rapidly by a blood transfusion or more gradually by iron replacement.

CASE 17

1. a) Hyperventilation (secondary)
   b) Partially compensated metabolic acidosis
2. Mesenteric ischaemia

What does the ABG tell us here? There is acidaemia due to a severe metabolic acidosis and the elevated lactate tells us it is a *lactic acidosis*. Lactic acid is produced by tissues receiving an insufficient supply of O_2 but oxygenation is normal (note the Pao_2 is appropriate for an Fio_2 of ~40%) and there are no clinical signs of shock (e.g. hypotension, cold peripheries), suggesting there is no generalised problem of O_2 delivery to tissues.

In fact, the source of lactic acid here is the bowel. The patient has mesenteric ischaemia, in which blood supply to the bowel wall is impaired due to occlusion of an artery by a thrombus or embolus. In the absence of an adequate blood supply, bowel tissue becomes hypoxic and must rely on anaerobic metabolism (producing lactate as a by-product).

Mesenteric ischaemia is a difficult diagnosis to make, as presenting symptoms, signs and routine investigations are all non-specific. The diagnosis should be considered in patients with minimal abdominal examination findings despite severe pain, especially in the presence of a lactic acidosis.

CASE 18

1. a) Hyperventilation (secondary)
   b) Severe metabolic acidosis with partial compensation
2. Anion gap = (141 + 4.6) − (96 + 6) = 43.6 (normal = 10–12)
3. Diabetic ketoacidosis

In diabetic ketoacidosis, severe insulin deficiency leads to hyperglycaemia and increased metabolism of fats. The breakdown of fats produces ketone bodies – small organic acids – which provide an alternative source of energy but can accumulate, leading to a profound metabolic acidosis. It is the ketone bodies that account for the raised anion gap.

In this case, the acidosis has overwhelmed not only the kidneys' ability to excrete an acid load but also respiratory compensatory mechanisms. There is therefore a severe and dangerous acidaemia despite near-maximal respiratory compensation.

An equally important problem in diabetic ketoacidosis is the profound osmotic diuresis resulting from hyperglycaemia that leads to severe dehydration and electrolyte loss.

CASE 19

1. a) Hyperventilation (secondary)
   b) Severe metabolic acidosis with partial compensation
2. 32
3. Yes

Methanol ingestion can be fatal in doses as small as 30 mL. Methanol is metabolised by the liver to produce formaldehyde and formic acid. Accumulation of formic acid leads to a profound acidosis with a raised anion gap. It also causes ocular toxicity and may result in permanent blindness.

$$\text{Anion gap} = (Na^+ \{136\} + K^+ \{4.5\}) - (Cl^- \{99\} + HCO_3^- \{9.5\})$$
$$= 140.5 - 108.5$$
$$= 32$$

Treatment for methanol poisoning is complex but often involves the administration of ethanol, which inhibits the conversion of methanol to its more toxic metabolites.

CASE 20

1. a) Slight hyperventilation (secondary)
   b) Compensated metabolic acidosis
2. Anion gap = $(137 + 3.0) - (109 + 18)$
   $$= 140 - 127$$
   $$= 13 \text{ (normal)}$$
3. Renal tubular acidosis (type 1)

The differential diagnosis of normal anion gap acidosis is relatively narrow, and in the absence of diarrhoeal symptoms, renal tubular acidosis (RTA) is the likely cause. The history of renal stones and associated hypokalaemia also supports the diagnosis.

In type 1 RTA, the kidneys fail to secrete H^+ into the urine in exchange for Na^+. This leads to excessive loss of HCO_3 in the urine, resulting in an acidosis. To maintain electroneutrality, extra Cl^- are retained (so it is a *hyperchloraemic* acidosis). Because Cl^- is a measured rather than unmeasured anion, there is no increase in the anion gap.

Type 1 RTA is often complicated by renal stones, as calcium tends to precipitate in alkaline urine, forming stones.

Hypokalaemia results because Na^+ are exchanged for K^+ instead of H^+.

CASE 21

1. a) Hyperventilation
   b) Compensated metabolic acidosis *or* metabolic acidosis with concomitant respiratory alkalosis
2. 27
3. Aspirin

Salicylate poisoning may cause both a primary respiratory alkalosis (direct stimulation of the respiratory centre) and a primary metabolic acidosis, as salicylate is an acid (it may also promote lactic acid formation). It is therefore not possible to ascertain confidently whether or not the hyperventilation is due to a primary effect of the aspirin or is a response to the metabolic acidosis.

The diagnosis would be confirmed in this instance by taking salicylate levels.

CASE 22

1. a) Mild hyperventilation (secondary)
   b) Compensated metabolic acidosis
2. Lactic acidosis, likely due to global tissue hypoperfusion
3. Elevated lactate

This patient with sepsis, most likely arising from the urinary tract, has a lactic acidosis, indicated by (i) the low HCO_3 (and high base deficit), (ii) a high anion gap (25.8 mmol/L) and (iii) an elevated lactate concentration. The probable cause of the high lactate is global tissue hypoperfusion.

Early measurement of lactate is a vital part of the initial assessment of sepsis and forms part of the '3-h bundle' in the surviving sepsis campaign guidelines.[1] ABG analysis is ideal for this purpose due to the rapid turnaround time and the additional information on gas exchange and overall acid–base status.

Although the observation chart for this patient shows a fall in blood pressure over the past few hours (and increasing tachycardia), the patient is not yet overtly hypotensive. Despite this, the elevated lactate indicates inadequate tissue perfusion and a risk of progression to septic shock. Indeed, even in the absence of hypotension, septic patients with a lactate level of 4 mmol/L or greater have a mortality rate of 30%. The decline in urine output over the preceding hours provides further evidence of impaired organ perfusion. Aggressive resuscitation is mandatory, with normalisation of lactate one of the key goals.

[1] See www.survivingsepsis.org

CASE 23

1. a) Hyperventilation (secondary)
   b) Severe metabolic acidosis with partial compensation
2. Hyponatraemia ($\downarrow$Na), hyperkalaemia ($\uparrow$K), hypoglycaemia ($\downarrow$glucose), raised lactate
3. Intravenous cortiocostcroids

This patient is likely to have adrenal insufficiency, a condition in which the adrenal glands fail to produce sufficient amounts of the hormone cortisol (and, in some cases, aldosterone). It often presents non-specifically with fatigue, malaise, anorexia and weight loss, and can be easily overlooked or misdiagnosed.

Lack of adrenal hormones causes salt and water depletion and loss of vascular tone, which, as in this case, may lead to dramatic circulatory collapse (acute adrenal crisis). The circulatory shock is the cause of the severe lactic acidosis.

Patients also have an inability to mobilise glucose reserves, hence the hypoglycaemia, and characteristic electrolyte abnormalities ($\downarrow$Na:$\uparrow$K).

In addition to basic life support and fluid resuscitation, the main intervention likely to improve this patient's condition is the administration of intravenous hydrocortisone.

CASE 24

1. a) Normal (i.e. satisfactory ventilation and oxygenation being achieved by bag and mask)
   b) Severe metabolic acidosis (uncompensated)
2. Prognosis: Very poor

In a cardiac arrest case, the ABG has several uses. It allows one to determine the adequacy of ventilation (in this case provided manually by bag and mask), to identify the presence of hyperkalaemia (one of the reversible causes of cardiac arrest) and may provide valuable prognostic information.

Here, despite the evident success of bag and mask ventilation in eliminating CO_2 and oxygenating blood, the patient has a profound lactic acidosis secondary to overwhelming tissue hypoxia. Although this may be multifactorial (e.g. the underlying disease process; hypoxaemia before bag and mask ventilation), the most important cause is inadequate tissue perfusion due to loss of cardiac function.

This patient has a grave prognosis. The level of acidosis is unlikely to be compatible with life and, given his unfavourable rhythm (an agonal rhythm does not respond to direct-current cardioversion and often signifies a 'dying heart'), age and co-morbidities, successful resuscitation is extremely unlikely.

CASE 25

1. a) Type 1 respiratory impairment (severe)
   b) Severe metabolic acidosis with partial compensation
2. 0.6–0.8
3. Acute pancreatitis

The diagnosis of acute pancreatitis is based on the history, examination findings and increased serum amylase level; the main use of the ABG is in helping to assess illness severity.

The severe lactic acidosis (high anion gap and increased lactate) indicates marked tissue hypoxia. The main cause is impaired blood supply to tissues due to circulatory collapse. This occurs as part of the systemic inflammatory response in pancreatitis and must be urgently corrected with aggressive fluid resuscitation ± vasopressor agents.

A Pao_2 of 10.8 with an Fio_2 of 0.6–0.8 implies severe respiratory impairment (see p. 16) and, together with chest X-ray appearances, suggests the development of acute respiratory distress syndrome (an inflammatory lung condition). Although Pao_2 is currently adequate, the patient may require ventilatory support if he deteriorates further or tires from the increased work of breathing.

Finally, the ABG also shows a high glucose and low calcium concentration – both of which are adverse prognostic factors in acute pancreatitis.

The patient should be transferred immediately to a critical care environment for intensive monitoring and supportive treatment.

CASE 26

1. a) Mild type 2 respiratory impairment (compensatory response)
   b) Compensated metabolic alkalosis
2. Electrolytes: Hypokalaemia ($\downarrow K^+$)
   Hyponatraemia ($\downarrow Na^+$)
   Hypochloraemia ($\downarrow Cl^-$)
3. Treatment: Fluid and electrolyte replacement

Vomiting causes loss of H^+ in gastric juice. The normal response of the kidneys to loss of H^+ is increased excretion of HCO_3^- to restore acid–base balance. *So why does this not happen?*

The reason is that persistent vomiting also leads to fluid, Na^+, Cl^- and K^+ depletion. In these circumstances, the overriding goal of the kidneys is salt and water retention.

Under the influence of a hormone called *aldosterone*, Na^+ are retained at the expense of either K^+ or H^+. If K^+ were plentiful, H^+ loss could be minimised, but K^+ is also in short supply so both are lost (worsening both the alkalosis and hypokalaemia).

Cl^- depletion also limits HCO_3^- excretion, as there must be enough negatively charged ions in blood to balance the positively charged ions (electroneutrality).

Thus, in this case, intravenous replacement of fluid and electrolytes (Na^+, Cl^- and K^+) would allow the kidneys to excrete more HCO_3^-, correcting the alkalosis.

CASE 27

1. a) Mild type 2 respiratory impairment (compensatory response)
   b) Metabolic alkalosis with partial compensation
2. Lower
3. Pyloric stenosis

Congenital pyloric stenosis is due to hypertrophy of the gastric outflow tract in the first 6 weeks of life. This obstructs flow between the stomach and duodenum, leading to projectile vomiting and inability to absorb nutrients.

As in the preceding case, persistent vomiting has caused significant loss of H^+, triggering a metabolic alkalosis. Again this is maintained because the associated fluid, Na^+, Cl^- and K^+, depletion prevents the kidneys from increasing HCO_3^- excretion. However, in this case, there is a severe alkalaemia for two reasons.

First, the metabolic alkalosis is more severe. This is mainly because of the greater duration of vomiting as well as because obstruction between the stomach and duodenum prevents HCO_3^- from the duodenum being lost in vomit.

Second, there is minimal respiratory compensation. Given the severe alkalaemia, one would predict a greater rise in $Pa\text{CO}_2$. This is probably explained by the child's distress, which provides an additional respiratory stimulus that blunts the compensatory response (i.e. a mild primary respiratory alkalosis).

CASE 28

1. a) Chronic compensated type 2 respiratory impairment
   b) Primary metabolic alkalosis, partially offset by primary respiratory acidosis with overall mild alkalaemia
2. Potassium supplementation or potassium-sparing diuretics

This patient has chronic type 2 respiratory failure due to advanced COPD. At first glance, it is tempting to ascribe her elevated HCO_3^- to metabolic compensation for the respiratory acidosis. However, there is an overall alkalaemia, indicating a primary metabolic alkalosis. By far, the most likely explanation for this is hypokalaemia due to aggressive diuretic therapy. Na^+ are retained in the distal portion of the kidney in exchange for either K^+ or H^+. In conditions of K^+ depletion, more H^+ are secreted in urine, resulting in a corresponding increase in HCO_3^-. The metabolic alkalaemia is unlikely to have major adverse clinical consequences but may be correctable with potassium supplementation or the addition of a potassium-sparing diuretic such as spironolactone or amiloride.

CASE 29

1. a) Appearance of severe type 1 respiratory impairment
   b) Normal acid–base status
2. Explanation: Venous sample

The ABG result suggests severe, life-threatening hypoxaemia, but the patient appears clinically well with only mild symptoms and no signs of major respiratory compromise. Moreover, there is a marked discrepancy between the So_2 as measured by pulse oximetry (99%) and that calculated on the ABG (74%). By far, the most likely explanation is that the sample was obtained from a vein rather than an artery. A repeat ABG should be performed.

It is important to ensure that an ABG sample is obtained from an artery before using it to assess the Pao_2. In addition to the aforementioned points, non-pulsatile flow and the need to draw back on the syringe at the time of sampling suggest venous blood.

CASE 30

1. a) Normal gas exchange
   b) Normal acid–base status
2. A – a gradient: 1.9 kPa/15 mmHg (normal)
3. Yes (must exclude pulmonary embolism)

This case is included to demonstrate the limitation of ABGs and the importance of considering the clinical context. The ABG is entirely normal but the patient is at high risk of pulmonary embolism, given her recent lower-limb orthopaedic surgery and subsequent immobility. Moreover, she has now developed sudden-onset pleuritic pain, breathlessness and tachycardia, unexplained by initial investigations.

While the finding of impaired oxygenation would have lent weight to a diagnosis of pulmonary embolism, a normal ABG result never excludes it. She therefore requires appropriate imaging (e.g. ventilation–perfusion scan or computed tomography pulmonary angiogram) to rule out this diagnosis.

$A - a$ gradient $= PAo_2 - Pao_2$
$\{(0.21 \times 93.8) - (4.9 \times 1.2)\} - 12.1$
$13.9 - 12.1$
$= 1.8$ kPa (normal $=< 2.6$ kPa)
OR
$\{(0.21 \times 713) - (37 \times 1.2)\} - 91$
$106 - 91$
$= 15$ mmHg (normal < 20 mmHg)

Index

N.B. Page numbers in italic denote material in Question & Answer section.

Page numbers followed by 'f' indicate figures, 't' indicate tables, and 'b' indicate boxes.